THE BrainWash

THEBrainWash

A Powerful, All-Natural Program to Protect Your
Brain Against Alzheimer's, Chronic Fatigue Syndrome,
Depression, Parkinson's, and Other Diseases

MICHELLE SCHOFFRO COOK

John Wiley & Sons Canada, Ltd.

National Library of Canada Cataloguing in Publication Data

Cook, Michelle Schoffro
      The brain wash : a powerful, all-natural program to
protect your brain against Alzheimer's, chronic fatigue syndrome, depression, Parkinson's and other brain diseases / Michelle Schoffro Cook.

Includes index.
ISBN-13: 978-0-470-83928-7

      1. Brain--Care and hygiene. I. Title.

QP376.C66 2007   612.8'2   C2006-906450-4

Production Credits:
Cover design: Mike Chan
Interior text design: Tegan Wallace
Cover Photo: Johnathan Kantor/Getty Images
Wiley Bicentennial Logo: Richard J. Pacifico
Printer: EPAC Book Services

John Wiley & Sons Canada, Ltd.
6045 Freemont Blvd.
Mississauga, Ontario
L5R 4J3

Printed in the United States of America

2 3 4 5 EPAC 13 12 11 10

The Brain Wash is dedicated to the memory of Roy Stickl,
and to the family he left behind.

It is also dedicated to all sufferers of brain disease. I wish you
tremendous health and happiness.

Table of

CONTENTS

Acknowledgements

I am blessed to be surrounded by so many incredible, kind, insightful, and supportive people in my work and my personal life. I would like to thank the many people who contributed to this book and who offered their support through the process of researching, writing, and editing:

To my soulmate and life partner, Curtis: I am eternally grateful for your love, support, and kindness. Thanks for always being there. Whatever our souls are made of, yours and mine are the same.

To Leah: You're a great editor and a wonderful person. It's been a tremendous pleasure working with you.

To my agent, Rick: Thanks for your ongoing belief in me and in my work over the years, as well as your many efforts to make this book possible.

To Jennifer and everyone else at Wiley: Thanks for believing in this book, for committing to it, and for helping to bring it to fruition.

To Claire Gerus: Thanks for your plentiful insights and assistance with developing this book concept.

To my parents: Thanks for believing in me and encouraging me along my writing path. I appreciate you as wonderful parents and friends.

To Michelle and David Harder at the Reynolds Hotel in beautiful Lillooet, BC, Canada: Thanks for your kindness and generosity in providing me with a quiet space in which to complete this book.

To Tutti Gould and Michelle Decary; for your contribution on homeopathy, a wonderful addition to this book.

To Juniper and Father Ron: Thanks for always looking out for me.

To my many wonderful and supportive friends and family members—thank you for your incredible friendship, love, support and insights, particularly Carri Drzyzga, DC; Anita Santos, DAc; and Cobi Slater, DNM.

Introduction

Your Brain Is at Risk

Consider how miraculous your body is. It is constantly changing. Your body regulates billions of different functions simultaneously…every single SECOND. Your skin is totally renewed every twenty-eight days. You have an entirely new heart in thirty days. Your lungs take seventy days to completely regenerate. What does this have to do with your brain, you may be wondering? Simple: the brain orchestrates almost every one of these miraculous achievements.

Arguably the most powerful organ in the body, the brain governs thoughts, moods, emotions, movement, speech, and every bodily function. Until recently, scientists believed that this mysterious organ was protected by an impermeable mechanism known as the "blood-brain barrier" that was understood to allow only nutrients to reach the brain without letting toxic chemicals in.

However, the most recent, cutting-edge research demonstrates that this barrier works on a lock-and-key type mechanism, wherein damaging chemicals can mimic vital nutrients and gain access to the brain. Recent discoveries show that this system allows many environmental toxins and heavy metals access to the delicate brain. Unfortunately, once these substances reach the brain, it can take decades to eliminate them—decades that can result in such substantial damage as inflammation and plaque build-up in the brain.

In light of this new understanding, a huge volume of new research links environmental toxins, chemicals… and altered fats in our food supply, and poor lifestyle choices to brain diseases like Alzheimer's, Parkinson's, depression, autism, and many others.

Consider one groundbreaking study entitled, *Toxic Nation: A Report on Pollution.* This study found that no matter where people live, how old they are or what they do for a living, they are contaminated with measurable levels of chemicals that are known to cause cancer, disrupt hormones, affect reproduction, cause respiratory problems, or impair neurological development. Canadians tested showed high levels of industrial pollutants, including lead, mercury, DDT, and PCBs. Astonishingly, the latter two have not been in commercial use for decades. Researchers found lead and mercury in the blood of ALL the subjects of this study, and Americans are no different. Every year the Environmental Protection Agency (EPA) performs a study of the chemicals found in human fat tissue samples. Chemicals like DDT continue to be found in one hundred percent of the tissue examined.

IT WON'T AFFECT ME

Today, nearly everyone is touched in some way by heart disease or cancer, often through a spouse, parent, family member, or friend. Perhaps we will personally experience one of these diseases. However, you may be shocked to learn that although these two primary killers will continue to take the lives of a record number of North Americans, there is another disease that will overshadow them. Scientists predict that within fifteen years, brain disease will kill or disable more North Americans than cancer and heart disease COMBINED!

In addition to the many disastrous personal and societal effects of brain disease, leading researchers estimate that the economic impact of this growing problem will be in excess of thirty billion dollars every year.

One in seven people currently live with brain disease, and almost 1.2 million people are diagnosed with brain disease in the United States alone every year. The number of people with Alzheimer's disease is expected to quadruple over the next fifty years—escalating from four to *fourteen* million. Another disease of the mind, attention deficit disorder (ADD), has increased five hundred percent in just fifty years!

That's where *The Brain Wash* comes in. Today, research has proven that genetic predisposition is only one predictor of brain disease. In fact, over one hundred studies show that environmental, nutritional, and lifestyle factors can play a significant role in initiating or accelerating brain disease. Researchers at Harvard School of Public Health and the Mount Sinai School of Medicine examined data on chemical toxicity and found, of the chemicals reviewed, over 200 have the capacity to damage the human brain. They add that chemical pollution may have already harmed the brains of millions of children worldwide and that one in six children has a developmental disability like autism, attention deficit hyperactivity disorder (ADH) and others. The authors of the study suggest that the widespread use of toxic chemicals in industry is a pandemic and that childhood exposures to these neurotoxins may be linked to increased risk of additional future brain diseases like Parkinson's. The lead scientists of this groundbreaking study, Philippe Grandjean, states: "You only have one chance to develop a brain." To that I would add, "You only have one chance to develop and protect a brain."

Fortunately scientists continue to prove that nutrition and lifestyle factors are able to protect the brain from damage.

Now you can follow the comprehensive and easy-to-implement suggestions in *The Brain Wash* to help prevent Alzheimer's, attention deficit disorder, autism, depression, Lou Gehrig's disease, multiple sclerosis, Parkinson's disease, and other brain disorders.

WHAT CAN I DO?

Scientists have discovered that certain foods and nutrients, eaten frequently and in specific doses, access the brain and actually escort toxins and metals out of the brain. The brain needs proper building blocks to create healthy cells. It needs oxygen, enzymes, nutrients, regular stimulation, and many other elements. *The Brain Wash* will show you how to protect your brain from destructive chemicals, created by industrial waste and synthetics, and help you avoid the vast array of brain disorders.

For the first time, *The Brain Wash* will teach you how to literally lock out brain-destroying toxins while letting in brain-building nutrients. You'll also learn about the worst brain-damaging substances (most are found in common foods and household products) so you can lessen your exposure. What's more, you'll master a step-by-step plan that is easy to incorporate into any lifestyle.

You are not powerless against the brain diseases many people believe are an inevitable part of aging. Now you can fight back and win.

The Brain Wash is a powerful health plan based on the most cutting-edge brain, nutrition, and healing research. *The Brain Wash* takes a truly holistic, mind-body-spirit approach to protecting your brain from damage, using foods, juices, herbs, and exercises to strengthen the brain. Meditation and breathing exercises found in the pages of this book will further assist in protecting against brain disease. The best of Western and Eastern healing approaches are combinded to help you improve memory, prevent disease, and even help reverse brain-related disorders.

I will discuss the most advanced brain research as well as ancient knowledge to help you protect your brain. You will learn about the many brain disorders that the average person is at risk of contracting: from Alzheimer's disease and Parkinson's to multiple sclerosis and depression. You will also discover the growing incidence of brain disorders affecting our children: from attention deficit disorder (ADD) to autism.

Research shows that staying slim, exercising, and eating a healthy diet helps to lower the risk of brain diseases like Alzheimer's.[1] Some of best medicine comes in the form of brilliantly coloured and delicious foods. *The Brain Wash* is based on the premise that you can take control of your life and your health.

Don't be a Victim of the SAD

After years of research into the nutrients required for brain health, I have come to the following conclusion: It is not possible to be emotionally stable and to maintain a healthy brain for life while eating the Standard American Diet (SAD).

A diet high in sugar and rapid blood sugar fluctuations is linked to depression, fatigue, confusion, and aggression. B-complex vitamins, which are essential for proper enzyme activity in the brain, are mostly devoid in the Standard American Diet. Adequate amounts of all essential amino acids are required for brain cells to be able to communicate properly, as well as for memory and hormonal balance. If brain cells do not communicate properly, almost any function in the body can be negatively influenced.

Your brain is sixty percent fat, so it should be no surprise that your body requires *healthy* fats to make healthy new brain cells. Without healthy essential fats, which are almost nonexistent in the Standard American Diet, the brain cannot replace worn or dying brain cells with healthy new ones.

Additionally, toxins in our food, water, air, and food supply that make their way into the body tend to settle in fatty tissues. In your body's wisdom, it attempts to keep toxins out of your blood so they cannot keep circulating and destroying cells and tissues. So, toxins end up in fat stores in your body. Unfortunately, the brain is one of those places. Later, I will explain how toxins gain access to the delicate brain and what you can do to stop them from doing so.

A study published in the journal *Food Review* showed that only four foods—canned tomatoes, fresh and frozen potatoes, iceberg lettuce, and onions—account for fifty percent of our total vegetable consumption in North America.[2] That is, of course, insufficient to maintain healthy brain cells. Phytonutrients, or plant nutrients, are found in all fresh fruits and vegetables, and are essential to a healthy body; yet, most people are not getting anywhere near adequate amounts. That worries me. It is with this in mind that I write *The Brain Wash* in an effort to help you understand that your food and lifestyle choices in large part determine your health.

YOU CAN TAKE CONTROL!

During the aging process, a type of protein called amyloid accumulates between our nerve cells (neurons). This protein build-up is accompanied by inflammation and oxidative damage, resulting in damaged cells and interrupted signals. If an excessive amount of proteins stick together, excessive cell damage may occur, causing memory loss, dementia, and other symptoms linked with brain disorders.

A diet packed with protective nutrients can slow the damage caused by amyloid build-up enough to fend off dementia. There is a growing body of research that shows foods, herbs, spices, and a healthy lifestyle may be your best protection against brain disease.

In addition, research shows that adequate amounts of key hormones and brain chemicals also are critical to brain health. These hormones and brain chemicals require plentiful amounts of particular nutrients found in many foods, herbs, and spices. Eating the foods discussed in *The Brain Wash* will help to protect your brain in numerous ways.

"For the majority of people, studies are showing you can probably slow down cognitive decline enough to escape disease altogether." [3]
~Greg Cole, PhD, associate director of the Alzheimer's Disease Research Center at the University of California, Los Angeles

As a doctor of natural medicine and a holistic nutritionist, I will expose the brain-killers in common foods and other hidden sources. I will also explore the latest research on healing foods like fish, berries, grapes, nuts, and spices, helping you to make better nutritional choices. As a holistic life coach, I will help you to understand how making healthier lifestyle choices can result in brain health throughout your lifetime. As a doctor of acupuncture and a Reiki Master, I will introduce you to Eastern therapies and techniques that can help keep your brain healthy.

There are thousands of studies proving the curative properties and potential of foods, nutrients, herbs and other natural medicines, and my purpose in writing *The Brain Wash* is to share with you the very best of these. You can make simple changes in your lifestyle habits, and you can learn to use natural medicines and healthy lifestyle choices to protect your brain against the onslaught of synthetic chemicals in our food, air, and water; to help ward off brain diseases; and to maximize your genetic potential.

We typically think of brain disease as merely the result of poor genes. That is only part of the story. Nature's rainbow-coloured medicines and other lifestyle factors play a critical role in determining the *expression* of genes, and whether a person develops disease symptoms or not.

I will also explore the latest research in botanical medicine and show how common herbs are offering tremendous promise, not only in brain protection, but also in strengthening memory in healthy individuals.

You will learn how easy it is to make simple changes to your diet that will have profound healing and protective effects. You will learn the essentials needed to make delicious and nutritious foods that are so good you'll forget about their brain-protecting qualities (but not for long: these foods will also help to strengthen your memory!).

Brain disease is not an inevitable part of aging, as many people believe. Arm yourself against brain disease with the most potent weapons—hose provided by Mother Nature herself.

chapter

1

Your Marvellous Brain in Action

"What lies before us, and what lies behind us, are tiny matters compared to what lies within us..."

~ Ralph Waldo Emerson

■ ■ ■ ■ ■ ■ ■

In chapter 1, "Your Marvellous Brain in Action," you will learn

- the fundamental workings of your brain;
- the difference between your brain and mind;
- how toxic chemicals get access to the brain and how they can cause damage;
- why it is important to consider the foods you put into your body; and
- how some critical nutrients found in foods, herbs, and nutritional supplements can help protect your brain from damage.

■ ■ ■ ■ ■ ■ ■

The average person's brain weighs only three pounds, yet it has over one hundred billion brain cells, which are called neurons. Neurons are connected to each other through synapses, which act like telephone lines between the brain cells.

If you took all the phones in the world and all the phone lines and wires, the trillions of messages per day would still not compare to the complexity or activity of a single human brain. And that only considers the wiring. As you'll soon discover, the human brain's capacity is so remarkable that no computer system on the planet could compare to it either.

Neurons are like on/off switches. When they are on, they send, receive, analyze, and coordinate information through electrical impulses that pass through them. When they are not being used, they remain in a resting state waiting for eventual use. Scientists estimate that the total amount of electrical charges generated by the brain at any given time is equivalent to a sixty-watt light bulb.

Each neuron has a long, wire-type substance called an axon that sends out hormones to generate the electrical charge between neurons. This electrical charge allows neurons to communicate. These hormones are called "transmitters" or "neurotransmitters." There are over a dozen types of neurotransmitters, and they each perform different functions, depending on what type of message the neuron is trying to send out. Some turn on functions in your body, while others stop bodily functions. Some of the main neurotransmitters are called dopamine, serotonin, epinephrine, and norepinephrine. Your brain tries to keep these hormones balanced to help you feel good and to maintain your health. When these hormones are imbalanced, illness or disease can form. You have your own ideal balance of neurotransmitters, which differs from someone else's. Actually, it's more accurate to state that you have a natural imbalance that helps to determine your likes, dislikes, skills and abilities, personality and character. Your particular neurotransmitter imbalance determines your thoughts, movements, pattern of breathing, and other functions in your body.

Synapses are constantly changing as a result of feedback from the environment. Naturally, over time synapses grow stronger through learning, while others weaken or disappear when they are not used. In other words, your brain starts to recognize which synapses appear to be needed and which ones don't. For example, your brain may initially set up all kinds of synapses linked to languages, but over time, because you're only developing skills in one language, synapses linked to learning new languages may start to disappear. That would be comparable to a telephone line dismantling the wiring and telephone poles on its own if it found that no one was using the line any longer—impossible! Yet the human brain does exactly that—every second of every day. This doesn't mean that you can't learn new languages or other skills down the road, but it would be easier if you continuously used these particular skills from childhood through adulthood.

Researcher William Greenough discovered a way to quickly increase the number of connections in animal brains by twenty-five percent simply by exposing the animals to what he called "an enriched environment." He states, "What we know from animals suggests that the harder you use your brain, whether it's thinking or exercising, the more in shape it's going to be."[1]

Greenough's research suggests more than just improved mental fitness through mental activity; it also suggests that by using your brain, your brain literally grows, not in girth, but in interconnectedness.

Greenough also found that there is an increase in brain capacity linked to further education. Although there is much research to suggest that educated people may be better able to ward off Alzheimer's, education alone is not enough to ensure improved brain function. For example, college graduates who have mentally inactive lives have fewer brain synapses than graduates who keep mentally active. Your education is less important than whether you continue to learn new things throughout your life. Your brain is designed for ongoing learning, and its health is dependent on it.

So you might think that the best example of the potential of the human brain would be found in someone with a post-doctoral education who maintained mental activity, even after she finished school. The reality is that an infant's brain is the best example of the immense potential for the human brain. By about eight months a baby's brain has about one thousand trillion connections, half of which will die off by the time the child is only ten, leaving five hundred trillion to last throughout the rest of her life. An infant's brain develops faster and better during the first few years than at any other time of life. A young child's brain thrives on feedback from its environment through sights, sounds, smells, tastes, and touches, and through interaction with others. Scientists believe that the extraordinary number of synapses in a baby's brain are formed to ensure that he will have sufficient "wiring" to be able to receive input from any environment he is born into.

A rich sensory environment is just as critical to an infant's development as adequate nutrition. Research shows that parents who talk to and read to their children from birth help to raise the child's IQ. More than that, parents help the infant develop the connections between brain cells that the child will use throughout life to learn languages, develop spatial skills, play a musical instrument, and for virtually every function or skill the child may need to develop in adulthood.

A Day in the Life of an Infant Brain

The brain goes through an enormous growth spurt in the first days of life by constructing trillions of connections between brain cells every day. These connections are then shaped through new experiences and will eventually become the basis for language, reasoning, ethical values, rationalization, and problem solving. Perhaps one of the most exciting discoveries about the brain is that it is not hard-wired; instead it uses the outside world to shape itself!

That is why external mental stimulation is so critical to the development of a child, and to the maintenance of pathways in the brain of an adult. You can always learn new things at any age, but the majority of the pathways in the brain will be determined during childhood. Says Ronald Kotulak, author of *Inside the Brain*: "In the crudest terms, the effect of environmental deprivation is just as physical as a blow on the head."[2] Lack of environmental stimulation, including being held, touched lovingly, and exposed to a variety of soothing sounds and visual stimuli, is one of the main ways in which the infant brain can be damaged.

Kotulak explains: "Without proper stimulation, the connections that allow brain cells to process sound, and thus language, become scrambled. They don't form the neat columns of cells that are so characteristic of the brain's architecture. According to Martha Pierson of the Baylor College of Medicine in Houston, such scrambling may cause childhood seizures, epilepsy, and language disorders. Pierson's remarkable experiments showed how experience, or the lack of it, can physically change the brain and cause mental disorders."[3]

Research indicates that while the brain never ceases to be able to grow, the years prior to twelve are the best for learning all sorts of things, including languages, music, art, and mathematics. Parents take note: this means that the early- and pre-school years are the most crucial years in determining life-long brain function! We will discuss great ways for you and your children to maximize the brain's potential in chapter 8.

In addition to the detrimental effects of experience deprivation, the brain can also be damaged from many other factors, including stress, nutritional deficiencies, poor food choices, alcohol, stroke, head trauma, and others, which you will learn in the coming chapters.

BRAIN COMMUNICATION

The brain sends and receives information in numerous ways. Some is received directly through vision and hearing, while other information, for example, is received as signals that help your arms and legs to move, pass through the spinal cord. Once signals reach the brain, they branch out across its surface (called the "grey matter" because the surface brain cells are grey in colour). Signals are then sent through the same channels to instruct the corresponding leg or arm muscles to move.

The brain is divided into two main sections: the left brain and the right brain. Each side handles different functions. The right brain controls the left side of your body, as well as visual tasks, artistic and creative functions, and collecting information, among many other functions. The left brain, in addition to controlling the right side of your body, also handles language, logic, rationalizing, and analysis of the information collected by the right brain.

Between these two sides of the brain is the corpus callosum, and it helps to ensure that the two sides of the brain communicate and work together.

THE BRAIN CAN HEAL

Scientists are discovering that your brain has the power to heal itself. The brain produces hormones and other natural chemicals that help sustain brain cells and preserve brain function. People with Alzheimer's, Parkinson's and other degenerative diseases demonstrate diminished levels of these critical hormones and brain chemicals.

Making sure that your body has all the essential nutrients required to create adequate hormone supply may be helpful in slowing the progression of such devastating diseases. The risk of Alzheimer's disease increases in women after menopause as their estrogen levels drop. Estrogen is showing itself to be a critical hormone in ensuring proper brain function. Even the male brain requires adequate estrogen. Dr. Frederick Naftolin, chief of obstetrics and gynecology at Yale University School of Medicine, discovered that an enzyme divides the sex hormone testosterone into its components, one of which is estrogen, to assist with healthy brain function.

Cell biologist Dominique Toran-Allerand showed that estrogen stimulates the production of the chemical called nerve growth factor, which functions exactly as its name would suggest: it helps ensure the growth and survival of brain and nerve cells. She also found that as estrogen production declines nerve growth factor also declines.[4]

Estrogen also prevents a decline in a brain chemical messenger called acetylcholine. Acetylcholine helps new memories to be imprinted in the brain.

In a healthy brain two main hormones, dopamine and acetylcholine, work together to regulate muscle activity. Acetylcholine helps muscles contract while dopamine softens the effects of acetylcholine. Acetylcholine has been found to be severely diminished in Alzheimer's patients, while dopamine is low in Parkinson's patients, resulting in muscles that stay too tightly contracted. I'll explain more about both of these disorders momentarily.

Other brain chemicals called neurotrophic factors also help to keep cells healthy and communicating properly with each other. If these factors decline or disappear altogether, the brain cells normally nourished by them shrivel.

There are many factors that can encourage a proper balance of these vital hormones and nutrients in your body and keep your brain working optimally. You will be learning about each in more detail as you read the chapters ahead, but first, let's take a look at the basic building blocks required by the brain.

THIS IS YOUR BRAIN ON THE STANDARD AMERICAN DIET (SAD)

So, what keeps this marvellous creation functioning? As you're probably aware, the brain needs adequate oxygen supplies. A loss of oxygen for six minutes could permanently damage the brain, and for seven minutes could result in death. Because you obtain oxygen through breathing, shallow breathing or inadequate exercise could lessen the amount of oxygen available to your brain. We'll discuss the importance of deep breathing exercises in chapter 8.

The brain is sixty percent fat and needs adequate supplies of high quality dietary fat to create healthy new brain cells. The brain also has need for a lot of energy. The brain uses about twenty percent of the entire energy supply of the body. That energy has to be supplied from your diet in the forms of complex carbohydrates and healthy sugars, yet the Standard American Diet, also aptly called SAD, does not include the right types of carbohydrates that your brain needs to keep it functioning healthily and to prevent illness over time. Your brain also needs amino acids from high quality protein to form the hormones called neurotransmitters to ensure that brain cells can communicate properly.

In addition, your diet needs to supply all the essential nutrients, like vitamins, minerals, and enzymes, to create and protect healthy brain cells that support the structure and functioning of your brain. A deficiency in any single nutrient can disrupt the health of the brain. This area of science, while still relatively young, is growing rapidly. Called nutritional neuroscience, it holds some of the greatest advancements for preventing brain disease and helping to support healthy brain functions. But you don't need to be a nutritional neuroscientist to understand or benefit from the advancements in research, as you'll soon discover in the coming chapters.

THE FLOWER LOSES ITS PETALS

When it comes to brain health, the dying brain cells are as important as the living ones. This may sound like a contradiction, but bear with me. There is an innate process in the brain that is something like a neurological death row. It is called *apoptosis* (Greek for a flower losing its petals) and is a process whereby the brain allots certain cells for destruction. Cells that have been damaged in some way, either by trauma, pathogens, toxins, or insufficient oxygen, are slated for death. They shrivel up and die quickly so no inflammation occurs, and then scavenger cells engulf the debris and recycle it to other living cells.

This programmed death process ensures that the remaining brain cells are healthy, strong, and vital, while damaged cells are prevented from causing further damage. How quickly or how slowly this process occurs determines the health of the brain. If the process occurs too quickly the brain will have limited capacity to create new cells to replace ones that are worn out and destroyed. On the other hand, if the process is too slow (or absent), the risk of cancer and other brain diseases increases. This is because damaged cells are allowed to live in the brain and may wreak havoc on other parts of the brain.

PROTECTING THE DELICATE BRAIN

The brain has a built-in mechanism to prevent unwanted substances from entering this delicate organ and potentially damaging brain cells, or at least that is what the "blood-brain barrier" does in theory. Nobel Prize winner Paul Ehrlich discovered this brain-protecting mechanism back in 1885. He injected blue dye into the bloodstream and observed that it stained almost every organ in the body, with the exception of the brain and spinal cord. He conducted additional studies in which he injected dye into cerebrospinal fluid, the fluid that helps to protect and nourish the brain, and found that this time the dye stained the brain. His research demonstrated the existence of what later became known as the "blood-brain barrier."

More recently, researchers have shown that this brain-protecting mechanism works on a lock-and-key-type mechanism. J. Robert Hatherhill, PhD, a leading toxicologist and professor of environmental toxicology, says it is more aptly termed the "BrainGate." He states that "it usually opens only to travellers with the proper keys. Those items that lack a key may approach the blood-brain barrier, but cannot pass through—hence the term BrainGate."[5] He adds:

Whether or not a molecule gains entry into the brain depends on several factors including its size and its ability to dissolve in fat. Because the tiny blood vessels or capillaries have cell membranes made of fats, agents that dissolve in fat pass relatively easily into the brain. Water-soluble molecules, such as proteins, hormones, antibiotics, and drugs used for cancer treatment, have a much more difficult time crossing the BrainGate. Those items that partially dissolve in both water and fat will slowly seep through the BrainGate, if given enough time.[6]

If you visualize a tollgate where different types of vehicles are trying to pass to the other side of the road, you'll have a good sense of how the BrainGate works. Similar to a tollgate where small cars, large cars, buses, transport trucks, and other types of vehicles all want to get to the other side of the toll station and continue on the road, the brain has numerous types of transport systems offering access to different types of substances, including glucose to fuel the brain, amino acids to form brain messengers, and other essential nutrients of all different shapes and sizes. Plus, in our modern age of pollution and adulterated foods, lots of other unnatural substances try to gain access to the brain.

Fat-soluble compounds can gain access to the brain so quickly that they could be completely eliminated from the blood in favour of the brain within a single pass through brain circulation, all of which could happen in a matter of mere minutes.

Hormones that are fat soluble, like estrogen, cross the blood-brain barrier readily, which explains why women taking estrogen replacement therapy often notice significant effects on their moods and other processes governed by the brain.

But what about important nutrients, like glucose, which the brain needs for fuel? Glucose doesn't dissolve in fat but needs access to the brain. The brain offers an alternative means of transportation to allow glucose to provide fuel to the brain. This system is a shuttle-type mechanism, whereby substances like glucose are carried directly to the brain. Potassium and sodium also quickly pass into the brain to allow for proper electrical activity. Of course, oxygen passes through quickly since the brain has high oxygen demands that must be satisfied for life.

Some toxic chemicals and heavy metals are able to masquerade as nutrients and gain access to the brain. In addition, substances that are commonly consumed or inhaled, like alcohol, caffeine, nicotine, or less common substances like amphetamines, cocaine, and heroin, readily cross over, as do many prescription and non-prescription drugs.

Amino acids must compete with each other for access to the brain. As a result, if one amino acid is found in high quantities in the blood, it can reduce the levels of other amino acids, which may result in serious brain imbalances. In chapter 4 you'll learn how adulterated amino acids like monosodium glutamate, or MSG for short, can have serious repercussions for the brain, particularly if they are consumed regularly.

As with any type of fat the brain is vulnerable to a process called "lipid peroxidation." That is a fancy term which basically means fats turning rancid. Similarly, if we eat poor quality fats, then they become part of the structure of the brain, creating an impaired blood-brain barrier. In chapter 6, you'll learn how harmful trans fats can disrupt the blood-brain barrier, thereby making the brain more susceptible to environmental toxins. Alternatively, consuming healthy fats can lessen the chances of suffering the ill-effects of exposure to toxins by protecting the blood-brain barrier.

Consuming healthy fats is not the only way you can protect the brain. Over one hundred studies show that environmental, nutritional, and lifestyle factors play a significant role in initiating or accelerating brain disease. Research even suggests that food can interact with genetic material to increase or decrease the risk of diseases, including genetic diseases. While this field is still in its infancy, it has demonstrated that what we eat affects our genes and our likelihood of suffering from a particular illness. This is empowering. It means that we can make choices to improve our genetic potential and protect our brain against brain disease at every meal and in the simplest of lifestyle choices.

Our food and lifestyle choices impact the rate at which we age, and the susceptibility of the brain to damage, by increasing or lessening free radicals throughout the body. Free radicals are charged molecules that destroy or damage cells in the body. They are involved with most of the symptoms we link with aging, like wrinkles, but also can cause immense damage to the brain. Nature's best defense against free radicals comes in the form of antioxidents. The good news is that through their antioxidant properties foods, herbs, and other natural medicines consistently prove effective at reducing the level of free radicals in the body.

So it may come as no surprise to learn that the brain has a high need for antioxidants. Nutrients that are classified as antioxidants are important to help the brain to prevent its fatty components from turning rancid, due to damage resulting from free radicals or environmental toxins, and to protect genetic material from damage that could otherwise initiate brain disease. Some of these important nutrients include vitamins C and E, natural plant pigments, and other critical nutrients known as carotenoids, lycopene, and bioflavonoids. Not to worry if that just sounds like chemical soup to you. I'll tell you where you can find these important nutrients and why you'll want to start consuming them.

Plus, I'll help you make great food and lifestyle choices that will help you on the road to brain health, whether you're interested in maintaining your brain's health, improving it, or preventing or treating brain disease. What's more, you'll learn how to put all your new knowledge together in chapter 8, "*The Brain Wash* Plan." It will guide you through five simple steps to help you make great food and lifestyle choices for long-term brain health.

PART

The Brain Killers

chapter

2

Heavy Metal and Your Brain

"Heavy metals cause serious health effects, including reduced growth and development, cancer, organ damage, nervous system damage, and in extreme cases, death."

~ Enviro Health Action

■ ■ ■ ■ ■ ■ ■

In chapter 2, "Heavy Metal and Your Brain," you will learn

- which heavy metals are linked to brain disease;
- how heavy metals impact your brain and your nervous system; and
- how you can minimize your exposure to heavy metals.

■ ■ ■ ■ ■ ■ ■

Heavy metal is a serious threat to the health of your brain. I'm not referring to the music of Ozzy Osbourne or Metallica, although too much headbanging has probably damaged more than a few brain cells. I'm referring to the metals found in your food, water, and air supply. You'll be amazed to learn where they lurk: in your favourite breakfast cereals, in flu and other vaccines, fish, popular processed foods, many calcium supplements, and common "medicines." Some heavy metals, such as mercury found in dental fillings, can become airborne (a process called "off-gassing") and be inhaled or absorbed through the skin in the same way lotions and creams are absorbed through contact. Experts estimate that at least twenty-five percent of the American population is likely to suffer from heavy metal poisoning. These heavy metals include cadmium, aluminum, lead, and mercury, all of which are increasingly being linked to brain disease.

This chapter will introduce you to the heavy metals that are linked to brain disease, explain how they impact the brain and nervous system, and teach you how you can minimize your exposure to heavy metals. If you have been exposed to heavy metals, or suspect high levels in your body, I will share valuable natural medicines and therapies later in this book to help you lessen your toxic load.

CADMIUM

Most people have never heard of this potentially damaging metal, yet it is toxic to every bodily system, in both children and adults, and can have serious repercussions in the brain.[1] Cadmium inhibits the formation and utilization of many enzymes and nutrients in the body, especially iron, a mineral that is essential for brain health. Cadmium also interferes with zinc and calcium absorption in the body and brain, making people more vulnerable to bone and immune system disorders, including malignant tumours.[2]

Henry A. Schroeder, MD, the former professor emeritus of physiology at Dartmouth Medical School and director of research at Brattleboro Memorial Hospital, administered high doses of cadmium to rats and found that it caused increased tension in their blood vessels. An increased level of blood vessel tension can heighten the risk of stroke. Other research revealed that, in humans, the urine of hypertensive patients contains up to forty percent more cadmium than the urine of people with normal blood pressure.

Symptoms of Cadmium Excess

- Anemia
- Decreased appetite
- Emphysema
- Hypertension
- Hypotension
- Kidney disease or damage
- Loss of sense of smell[3]

It is possible to have a heavy metal excess without having all of the symptoms outlined in the lists provided throughout this chapter. Since many symptoms can also indicate other health concerns, it is best to consult a physician if you suspect heavy metal toxicity of any kind. There are laboratory tests that can be done to determine the levels of heavy metals in the body. While traditional doctors may be able to offer blood tests, these results are usually only of value in identifying recent or acute exposures. Some doctors of natural medicine offer hair analysis, which better identifies the levels that may have settled into the body's tissues, or urine analysis, which helps to identify the amount of metals your body is attempting to excrete.

Where Does Cadmium Hide?

Cadmium is found in numerous places in society. Its primary uses are industrial in nature, so you'll find it in batteries and electronics. Sewage sludge, which is often used as commercial fertilizer for crops, also contains high levels of the brain- and kidney-damaging heavy metal. Studies in Sweden indicate an increase in cadmium in crops over time.[4] This has led to the discovery of cadmium in some cereal grains, and root and leafy vegetable crops. Plants tend to absorb cadmium in higher levels than other metals.

Cadmium is also found in cigarette smoke, which is ingested either through smoking or exposure to second-hand smoke. According to environmental toxicologist J. Robert Hatherhill, PhD, smoking one pack of cigarettes per day exposes your body to ten times more cadmium than a person's body can handle in a single day.[5]

Potential Sources of Cadmium

- Automobile seat covers
- Black rubber
- Burned motor oil
- Ceramics
- Cigarettes
- Drinking water

- Evaporated milk
- Fertilizers (superphosphates)
- Floor coverings
- Fungicides (including those sprayed on apples, tobacco, and potatoes)
- Furniture
- Paint pigments
- Pesticides
- Refined wheat flour
- Rubber tires
- Sewage sludge
- Silver polish
- Soft drinks from vending machines with cadmium in the pipes[6]

Iron and steel manufacturing distributes huge amounts of cadmium into the environment. Yet no records are kept on the cadmium content of metallic scrap or cadmium released as vapour into the environment. Dr. Richard Casdorph and Dr. Morton Walker, two leading researchers on heavy metals, believe that changing environmental requirements in just these two areas would save many people from Alzheimer's disease.[7]

Aluminum

Although not strictly a heavy metal, aluminum is the most abundant metal on the planet. It is naturally found in air, food, soil, and water. Our bodies can excrete small amounts of aluminum without damage. Some experts estimate that a daily allowance of about twenty milligrams of aluminum poses no threat to health. But our modern-day exposure to aluminum often exceeds this amount, sometimes substantially, and with potentially serious consequences.

Aluminum is a known neurotoxic agent linked to Alzheimer's disease. Forty years ago, scientists injected aluminum into the brains of rabbits and made a startling discovery: aluminum triggered the formation of neurofibrillary tangles, the same type found in

Alzheimer's disease.[8] This caused researchers to examine diseased human brains.

Aluminum can cross the blood-brain barrier and cause nerve cell death. Once aluminum enters into the brain, it promotes inflammation by causing the formation of brain-damaging free radicals[9] and induces numerous toxic reactions, including the disruption of calcium control.[10] Aluminum makes its way into the brain by essentially impersonating iron, thereby tricking the brain into allowing it to cross the blood-brain barrier.[11]

There are abnormally high concentrations of the metal aluminum in the brains of people diagnosed with Alzheimer's.[12] Some studies indicate that the brains of Alzheimer's patients contain thirty times the levels of aluminum of their healthy counterparts.[13] There is still debate as to whether aluminum causes Alzheimer's, or if the accumulation of aluminum is the result of the disease, but it is known that aluminum is so toxic to the brain that it interrupts over fifty brain chemical reactions, and its relationship to Alzheimer's is undeniable.[14]

Additional studies are being done to better understand the toxic effects of elevated exposure to aluminium, and so far the results are frightening. Not only has aluminium been shown to have ties to Alzheimer's, but also to the increasing incidence of Parkinson's disease.[15]

Symptoms of Aluminum Excess

- Belching accompanied by head colds
- Colic
- Constipation accompanied by throbbing headaches
- Convulsions
- Cravings for meat
- Excessive perspiration
- Gastrointestinal irritation
- Indigestion caused by potatoes
- Loss of taste
- Nausea

- Numbness, stiffness, or loss of sensation in arms/legs
- Poor or failing memory
- Rickets
- Rough skin
- Stitching or burning pain in head with dizziness, relieved by eating [16]

Similar to cadmium, aluminum excess can occur in the body without having all of the above symptoms. It is best to ask your doctor to test for aluminum toxicity if you suspect it may be a concern.

Where Does Aluminium Hide?

Aluminum is primarily found in certain food items, like those containing baking soda or baking powder, which means most baked goods. It is also hidden in common personal care products like creams, deodorants and shampoo. But, you may be surprised to learn that it is even found in some nutritional supplements.

Potential Sources of Aluminum

- Baby formula
- Baked goods and processed foods
- Binding agents in many pharmaceutical drugs
- Commonly used medications and over-the-counter antacids
- Deodorants
- Food storage wrap like foil and pie plates
- Municipal water supplies
- Pots and pans
- Shampoo
- Skin creams
- Vitamin C supplements

Shampoo and skin cream may contain aluminum that can be absorbed through your skin. This is especially true of dandruff shampoo.

If it contains either magnesium aluminum silicate or aluminum lauryl sulphate, the product should be avoided altogether. Brands that don't list the ingredients on the label should also be avoided.

Cooking in aluminum pots and pans, or using aluminum pie plates or foil can cause aluminum to leach into your food. A study conducted by the University of Cincinnati Medical Center indicated that if tomatoes are cooked in an aluminum container, the aluminum content per serving increases by two to four milligrams.[17]

▦ ▦ ▦ ▦ ▦ ▦ ▦

Antacids and Aluminium

Some antacids contain up to two hundred milligrams of aluminum in a single tablet. Yet, the commercials for these products tell us that they are an excellent source of calcium and encourage us to pop the potentially brain-damaging tablets like candy. Regular users of antacids may be ingesting up to four grams (or four thousand milligrams or two hundred times the maximum daily allowance) of aluminum daily.

Some antacids that may contain aluminium:

Generic Name: aluminum hydroxide (with magnesium carbonate, or magnesium hydroxide, magnesium hydroxide and simethicone, or magnesium trisilicate).
Brand Names: Gaviscon, Aludrox, Di-Gel, Gelusil, Maalox, Magalox, Mylanta.
Rolaids, Pepto-Bismol, and Remegel.[18]

▦ ▦ ▦ ▦ ▦ ▦ ▦

Your food and water may also contain excessive aluminum. This metal is used as an emulsifying agent, particularly in foods like processed cheeses (including Kraft and Cracker Barrel), cookies (including Oreos), packaged cereals, canned foods, pancake and cake mixes, self-rising flour, prepared dough, non-dairy creamers, pickles, iodised table salt, gelatin desserts, including every child's favourite Jell-O, some brands of baking soda and baking powder (and therefore, any foods made with them), and even nutritional supplements. Worse, aluminum is even added to many brands of baby formula.

A study from researchers at the University of Toronto discovered a 250 percent increased risk of Alzheimer's disease in people whose drinking water contained high levels of aluminum for more than ten years.

LEAD

Some researchers attribute the fall of the Roman Empire to the heavy metal lead. Romans used lead materials in their food storage vessels and to line the aqueducts used for transporting water. Since lead is a known neurotoxin that is proven to affect mental performance, researchers believe that ancient Romans lost some of their mental capacities and abilities to make intelligent choices, thereby causing their own demise. Whether or not you accept this theory, it is easy to understand why lead is a serious threat to health.

Lead crosses the blood-brain barrier and can cause senile dementia and Alzheimer's, and learning disabilities and such as attention deficit disorder and aggressive behaviours. Significant research shows that lead poisoning affects the pre-frontal cortex of the brain, the part that governs impulse behaviour, and may cause someone to react violently if disrupted. Due to the persistent nature of lead, this heavy metal tends to build up in our bodies over time, and toxic effects may be slow to develop yet may last throughout a person's lifetime.[19]

Some of the harmful effects of lead include low birth weight, increased childhood mortality, and psychiatric disorders. Lead also disrupts calcium metabolism and various brain messengers critical for controlling emotions, learning, and memory. Lead blocks the formation of hormones like dopamine and serotonin. Mental functions such as impulse control and managing violent behaviours depend on adequate production of both of these hormones. At least seven studies have shown that violent criminals have elevated levels of lead, cadmium, manganese, mercury, and other metals compared with prisoners who are not violent. Lead is also linked with progressive mental decline.

Adults retain between five and fifteen percent of the lead they ingest. Children can absorb over forty percent of the lead they ingest. This is a serious concern. Infants and children in a rapid growth phase absorb more heavy metals such as lead than do adults.

Heavy Metals and Milk

Lead travels through the body and eventually gets to the bones and stays there for decades or more. Since lead disrupts calcium uptake in the body, it may be easy to assume that a person who has been exposed to lead should drink more milk. Not true. Studies show that milk consumption actually increases lead and cadmium absorption. The main protein in milk, casein, has been shown to increase lead levels in the brains, livers, and kidneys of animals. Researchers have not determined why this happens, but it is possible that heavy metals piggyback on the amino acids in milk to get access to the brain. Milk fat also increases uptake of lead and other environmental pollutants.[20] Saturated butterfat has shown the most dramatic increase in lead uptake. Researchers are attempting to understand why this happens, but most likely lead also piggybacks on the fat molecules to gain access to the brain. Metals and other toxins have an affinity for fats, while the brain has particularly high fat needs. That combination can have disastrous consequences when toxins are present.

Additionally, lactose (milk sugar) enables greater absorption of lead in your body than do other types of dietary sugars. When it comes to milk and dairy products, it really is a case of "three strikes and you're out." In the presence of lead and other environmental toxins, which all of us are subject to, milk does nothing but harm the body.

Symptoms of Lead Excess

- Abdominal discomfort
- Anxiety or irritability
- Constipation
- Convulsions or seizures
- Cramps or abdominal aches

- Dizziness
- Fatigue
- Hand tremors
- Hyperactivity in children
- Impaired long-term memory
- Lack of ambition, apathy, or depression
- Listlessness
- Nervousness or restlessness
- Pallor
- Paralysis
- Poor coordination
- Sallow complexion or greyish, greenish, or yellowish tint to skin
- Susceptibility to colds, flu, or infections
- Vomiting
- Weakness[21]

Since the above symptoms can also indicate other health concerns, it is best to consult a physician if you suspect heavy metal toxicity of any kind, including lead. There are laboratory tests that physicians can conduct to determine lead levels in your body.

Potential Sources of Lead

- Canned food
- Ceramic dishes
- Cigarette smoke
- Coloured, glossy newsprint
- Leaded candle wicks
- Lead Paint
- Lead water pipes
- Municipal water supplies
- Refined chocolate
- Soil
- Soldered water pipes
- Vehicle emissions

There are many sources of lead in the environment, including vehicle emissions (although leaded gasoline has been prohibited from use in Canada since 1990, gasoline emissions are still a source of lead in the environment), cigarette smoke, water from pipes with solder, food in tins with soldered seals, food wrappings, coloured glossy newsprint, soil, leaded wicks in candles, and water. Rice and vegetables cooked in contaminated water have been shown to absorb eighty percent of the lead.[22]

Recent research also found that processed chocolate may be contaminated with extremely high quantities of lead. Originally it was assumed that cacao plants were tainted by leaded gasoline, however, a team of researchers found that lead levels in processed chocolate are sixty times higher than in other forms of chocolate. That doesn't mean you have to give up chocolate altogether. Getting your chocolate in the form of organic cocoa is best.

Lead and Your Home

Part of what makes lead particularly dangerous is its potential to be odourless, tasteless, and invisible. But there is much you can do to reduce your lead exposure, starting with knowing the sources within your own home. For example, did you know that the plastic insulation of wires contains lead, and that imported vinyl mini-blinds often have lead-containing additives to add strength and colour stability? Even the dust released from these blinds contains high levels of lead! Imported ceramic dishes are another possible source of lead contamination in your home. The lead can leach into foods or liquids, particularly if the foods are acidic. Storing or cooking in ceramic dishes containing lead increases the likelihood of contamination.

Lead is commonly found in homes through paint, but it lurks in other areas as well, particularly in tap water. According to the United States Environmental Protection Agency (EPA), approximately twenty percent of public water systems, serving thirty-two million people, were found to have lead levels exceeding their safety standard of fifteen parts per billion.

According to the company Pro-Lab Inc., your water may be contaminated with lead if your home has

1. Lead pipes and/or lead connectors from the water main;
2. Copper pipes with lead solder;
3. Soft water—a water softener can contribute to the corrosiveness of the water and, if used, should not be connected to lead pipes or pipes that contain lead solder leading to drinking water taps.

Additionally, the longer water has been sitting in your home's pipes, the more lead it may contain. Lead-contaminated water from lead pipes and fixtures contributes to lead poisoning in over forty million homes.[23] Your home's age is a contributing factor. If the plumbing was installed prior to 1930, it most likely has lead pipes. If the plumbing was installed or replaced prior to 1988, it may contain lead solder.

There are lead test kits for water testing or surface testing. Some water kits will test to levels as low as one part per billion for water (EPA standards are fifteen parts per billion). Surface tests are available for testing lead levels to as low as five parts per million.

As for lead paint, most homes built prior to 1978 may contain paint with high levels of lead. Lead-based paint was used on walls, ceilings, wood, furniture (including baby cribs), window frames, children's toys, and floors, and these items pose a very real health risk. According to Pro-Lab Inc., ingesting lead paint and breathing lead dust from old paint is the main contributor for lead poisoning, which causes brain damage and affects over two hundred thousand children every year.

Even short-term exposure to lead is estimated to drop a child's IQ three points for every ten micrograms/decilitre of lead in his or her blood. If the exposure goes undetected, a child may suffer permanent damage, resulting in problems ranging from learning disabilities to severe mental disability or even death. Children, especially those under seven years, are more susceptible to damage from lead because their developing bodies absorb the toxic metal at four times the rate of an adult. Pregnant women are also at greater risk, as are their unborn babies.

Before you start the renovations to remove lead, keep in mind that renovation projects can create high levels of paint dust and therefore lead dust. It is important to consult a professional skilled in lead paint removal or encapsulation.

Calcium Supplements, Antacids, and Lead

Many calcium supplements contain significant amounts of lead. In a study published in the *Journal of the American Medical Association*, three Florida researchers analyzed the lead content in twenty-one calcium supplements, available without a prescription and popularly used, and found that eight had measurable lead content ranging from 1.74 milligrams to 3.43 milligrams in a fifteen hundred milligram dose. Fifteen hundred milligrams of calcium is the daily-recommended dose for people suffering from osteoporosis.[24]

Most manufacturers of calcium supplements claim that all calcium will have some lead since they are found together in nature. While there is some truth to the claim, the levels of lead should not be detectable. In a study cited by J. Robert Hatherhill, PhD, in *The BrainGate*, lead was found in the following brands of calcium supplements: Source Naturals, GNC, Country Life, Rainbow, TwinLab, Longs, Savon, Your Life, Schiff, Os-Cal, Jarrow, Caltrate, Walgreens, Spring Valley, Solgar, Nature Made, Target, Posture-D, and Tums.

Dr. Hatherhill also indicates that detectable levels of lead have been identified in various brands of antacids, including: Di-Gel, Rolaids, Mylanta, and Childen's Mylanta.

MERCURY

The heavy metal, mercury, shares a characteristic with the ancient Greek mythological figure Mercury, the god of speed. The heavy metal also exhibits speed in its ability to gain access to the delicate brain.

Drs. Mercola and Klinghardt state, "Mercury exposure and toxicity is a prevalent and significant public health threat."[25]

Mercury is a well-established neurotoxin.[26] As I mentioned earlier, a neurotoxin is a substance that is damaging to the brain and nervous system. In the case of mercury, it has been connected with brain diseases like Alzheimer's.[27] Research shows that people with Alzheimer's disease often have blood levels of mercury up to three times higher than people who are not suffering from the disease.[28]

In another study, researchers added small amounts of mercury to cultured neurons in a laboratory and found seven cell features that are used in the diagnosis of Alzheimer's disease.[29]

Mercury is quite resistant once it makes its way into our bodies, and over time, can be damaging to nerve and brain cells. The symptoms of mercury excess, according to neurologist, Dr. David Perlmutter, are similar to severe brain aging, because in a sense mercury is aging the brain. In his book, *The Better Brain Book*, Dr. Perlmutter states that "mercury does its dirty work by promoting free radical production and inflammation; this is the same process that causes normal brain degeneration, but mercury does it much faster."[30] Essentially, mercury exposure speeds the aging of the brain.

This is especially true in infants. Because they are unable to excrete mercury, it accumulates in the brain cells, nerves, gut, and liver, and can cause the symptoms of poisoning.[31]

Numerous studies demonstrate that once mercury makes its way into the central nervous system (CNS), it causes psychological, neurological, and immunological problems in humans. Unfortunately, due to the strong binds created between mercury and the CNS, it can be hard to eliminate. Other studies show that mercury is taken up by all nerve endings and rapidly transported inside the axon of the nerves to the spinal cord and brainstem. Experts estimate that unless mercury is actively removed, it has a half-life between fifteen and thirty years in the CNS, which means it takes between fifteen and thirty years for only half of the mercury to be eliminated if more active mercury elimination attempts are not undertaken.[32]

Research links mercury exposure to heart arrhythmias and disorders. It has also been associated with neurological problems like tremors, insomnia, polyneuropathy (a degenerative disease of the nerves caused by toxins), paresthesias (prickling or tingling sensations of the nerves usually resulting from nerve damage), emotional instability or changeability, irritability, personality changes, headaches, weakness, blurred vision, dysarthria (difficulty communicating due to central nervous system disease), slowed mental response, and unsteady mobility."[33]

Symptoms of Mercury Excess

- Allergic tendencies
- Confusion
- Convulsions
- Depression or uncontrollable crying
- Diabetes
- Difficulty chewing or swallowing
- Facial and back pain
- Fatigue
- Food cravings
- High blood pressure
- Inflamed gums
- Irritability
- Loss of ability to speak
- Loss of appetite
- Loss of self-confidence
- Memory loss
- Mental disturbances or personality changes
- Metallic taste in the mouth
- Poor memory
- Tremors or poor coordination[34]

While it is possible to experience no symptoms of mercury toxicity, typically one or more of the above symptoms will be present. If you have poor health, or believe you have had exposure to mercury, it is best to be tested to determine your body's mercury levels, especially considering the serious nature of this metal in the body.

Children and fetuses are at greatest risk of suffering from the dire consequences of excess mercury exposure. If their nervous systems and brains are exposed to mercury during development, the damage may be far worse than for a fully developed adult.

Some experts believe mercury exposure may trigger autism in children. Dr. Perlmutter indicates that each year in the United States as many as three hundred thousand babies are at risk of brain damage from mercury exposure in the womb.[35]

The Centers for Disease Control and Prevention (CDC) released a study indicating that five percent of all American women of childbearing age are believed to have mercury levels in their blood in excess of the EPA's safety threshold. An additional five percent have levels that are just below the threshold.

A study by a physician in San Francisco found that sixteen percent of all people tested had mercury levels that were substantially higher than those deemed safe by the United States Environmental Protection Agency, which is five parts per billion.[36] You may also recall the earlier Canadian study that found mercury in the blood of one hundred percent of the people tested.

Primary Sources of Mercury

- Dental fillings
- Fish
- Immunizations

Mercury is emitted into the environment from coal-fired power plants, through medical waste incinerators, and trash incinerators. Once mercury makes its way into the air, it falls as rain into oceans, lakes, rivers, and streams. Bacteria in the water break the mercury down into an organic form called methyl mercury, which is highly toxic. We may ingest this mercury through our water supply or from the fish found in these mercury-laden waters. A diet high in fish, especially halibut, king mackerel, shark, swordfish, tilefish, white albacore tuna (both canned and fresh), and farmed salmon, makes it easy to exceed the

EPA's allowable amount of mercury in the body. As a result, the Food and Drug Administration (FDA) issued a warning advising pregnant women not to eat the fish with the highest levels of mercury because of the potential harm to their fetuses.

Fish containing the lowest levels of mercury include sardines, haddock, wild or Pacific salmon, and tilapia.

Food sources are not the only culprits. There are two other common sources of mercury.

It's All in Your Head

One of the worst sources of mercury sits right beneath your nose. All those silvery-metallic dental fillings known as amalgams in your mouth contain mercury.

In the *Journal of Nutritional and Environmental Medicine*, Dr. Mercola and Dr. Klinghardt state that people with amalgam fillings exceed all occupational exposure allowances of mercury in all European and North American countries. Adults with four or more amalgams run a significant health risk from the amalgam, while in children, as few as two amalgams will contribute to health problems.

According to Mercola and Klinghardt, a single dental amalgam with a surface area of 0.4 square centimetres is estimated to release up to fifteen micrograms of mercury per day, primarily through mechanical wear and evaporation.[37]

The average person with four amalgam fillings will absorb up to 120 micrograms of mercury per day, just from their fillings. Compare that with the daily estimates of mercury absorption from fish and seafood, which is 2.3 micrograms, and from all other foods, air, and water is 0.3 micrograms per day.

Amalgams—also called "silver" fillings—are usually made up of fifty percent mercury, thirty-five percent silver, nine percent tin, six percent copper, and a trace of zinc.

More than one hundred million mercury fillings are placed each year in the United States, as over ninety percent of dentists still use them for restoring teeth. Mercury escapes continuously for the duration the filling is left in the teeth. It escapes primarily in the form of vapour ions but also as abraded particles. Chewing, brushing, and ingesting hot fluids and foods stimulates this release.[38]

Because of the high mercury exposure dental amalgams can cause, countries like Germany, Sweden, and Denmark have already started to severely restrict the use of amalgams. An advocacy group called Citizens for Mercury Relief started an international petition, Ban Mercury In Teeth Everywhere (BITE). The group currently has signatures from citizens in over forty countries and is taking its petition to international dental assocations.

Approximately eighty percent of American adults have mercury amalgams in their teeth.[39] The American Dental Association claims that mercury amalgams are safe and that mercury cannot escape once it is sealed in an amalgam. But the scientific literature begs to differ.

Numerous studies demonstrate that amalgam fillings are linked with many diseases, including: Alzheimer's, autoimmune disorders, kidney dysfunctions, infertility, polycystic ovary syndrome, neurotransmitter imbalances, food allergies, multiple sclerosis, thyroid problems, and impaired immune systems.[40] Other studies show that people with many amalgams have an increase in the occurrence of antibiotic-resistant bacteria in their bodies.

Mercola and Klinghart state, "Animal studies show that...mercury released from ideally placed amalgam fillings appear quickly in the kidneys, brain, and wall of the intestines."[41]

The concentration of mercury vapor in the oral cavity of a patient with many amalgam fillings reaches fifty thousand parts per million or higher, as detected by the Jerome mercury vapour meter and shown on CBS television's *60 Minutes* in 1990. Mercury vapours are created by chewing, resulting in polluted air that a person then inhales and exhales. Tekran Instruments Corporation of Toronto, Canada, conducted a study at an environmental conference in Fredericton, New Brunswick, in September 1998 showing the mercury vapour levels in the air in the hotel hosting the conference doubled from five parts per million to ten parts per million during coffee breaks. Tekran identified mercury emissions from dental fillings, increased by heat from hot coffee, as the source of this toxic air. This means that people who have dental amalgam are the largest mercury polluters indoors.[42]

There is no controversy over mercury being a toxic material that has significant neurological and other serious health effects. There is, however, controversy stemming from dental associations' claims versus a growing body of scientific evidence that mercury amalgams pose a threat to health. The American Dental Association claims that amalgams are safe and that mercury in them does not pose a health threat. The Canadian Dental Association claims that there is no scientific evidence linking illness to mercury fillings. The US government's own National Health and Nutritional Exam Survey (NHANES III) database shows that people with more than four dental fillings (the average number of amalgams at the time the survey was done) have higher rates of certain illnesses, such as multiple sclerosis, compared to the general population.

In most places in North America, employees exposed to mercury vapour in the workplace have legislation protecting them. Companies are obligated to provide mercury safety equipment, perform regular monitoring of air quality, regularly test workers for mercury exposure, and reduce mercury use as much as possible using alternative material options. Dentists are exempt from any of these requirements. As an example, in Ontario the exemption is specifically contained in the Revised Rules and Regulations Governing Mercury.

In the safety data sheet for dental amalgams provided by Dentsply Caulk, Milford, Delaware, the company lists medical conditions generally aggravated by mercury exposure as: "chronic respiratory disease, nervous system disorders, and kidney disease." The safety data sheet also advises people to "always keep mercury stored in a sealed container away from heat" and "wear appropriate protective clothing to prevent any possibility of skin contact with this substance."[43] The Environmental Protection Agency and the United States military has declared the amalgams removed from teeth are toxic waste. If amalgams removed from the human body are considered toxic waste, why are we still placing them in our bodies? That's a question that government bodies seem to avoid.

Dentists have been asked to perform numerous cognitive and behavioural tests and the results have been compared with members of the general population. In one study, the dentists had fourteen percent worse scores in memory, coordination, motor speed, and concentration. In other studies, the dentists have shown higher rates of cancer, depression, irritability, chronic fatigue, headaches, tremors, arthritis, infertility, and miscarriages.

A study based in the United Kingdom, and published in the *Occupational and Environmental Medicine Journal*, examined the health effects of mercury on dentists. This study found that 180 dentists had on average four times the urinary mercury excretion levels of 180 people in the control group. Also, dentists were significantly more likely than control subjects to have had disorders of the kidneys and memory disturbances.[44]

Both methylmercury and mercury vapours from dental amalgams have been proven to find their way into the brain. Methylmercury can bind to an amino acid from protein to create a complex that resembles another amino acid, thereby tricking the brain. Once mercury finds its way into the brain, numerous toxic processes take place, including the depletion of essential antioxidants that protect the brain, subsequent stress on the brain, and the blocked formation of an important brain messenger called "acetylcholine." Acetylcholine transmits messages that regulate nerve-muscle activity and memory through the brain and nervous system.

The direct toxicity of mercury is not the only problem with its use in dentistry. Metal tooth restorations also produce electrogalvanic effects. In other words, mercury amalgams create a battery-like effect in the mouth because of the conductibility of saliva. Mercola and Klinghart state that: "the electrical current causes metal ions to go into solution at a much higher rate, thereby increasing the exposure to mercury vapour and mercury ions many times. Gold placed in the vicinity of an amalgam restoration produces a ten-fold increase in the release of mercury."[45]

The existence of mercury in the body presents another health threat, according to Dr. Perlmutter. "If you are constantly challenging your body with a high toxic load, your brain is likely to be spending all its time fighting free radicals as opposed to maintaining and repairing brain cells. As a result, whatever memory, concentration, or other cognitive problems you are having now will only get worse."[46]

While urine and feces are the main excretory pathways of metallic and inorganic mercury in humans, the most important element of a mercury elimination program is to remove dental amalgams. However, be forewarned that removal of mercury fillings without adequate precautionary measures can also cause the release of sizable amounts of mercury into your blood, which could, in turn, find its way into your brain. It is essential to find a highly skilled dentist with specialized training in the removal of mercury fillings, and to work with a holistic doctor skilled in mercury detoxification.

Preserving Health?

Mercury is used as a preservative, called thimerosal, in vaccines. With the rapidly rising incidence of autism in Canada and the United States, thimerosal use is hotly debated amongst health professionals. Thimerosal was used in almost all vaccines until recently. Even now, it is used in many vaccines for children and adults. Of the vaccines that still contain mercury, the flu vaccine is the biggest concern, according to Dr. David Ayoub, the director of the Prairie Collaborative for Immunization.

About eighty percent of flu vaccines contain as much as twenty-five micrograms of mercury per dose. The Environmental Protection Agency's safe limit for mercury exposure is 0.1 micrograms per kilogram, so only a 550-pound person could receive a flu vaccine and fall within the EPA's safe exposure limits for mercury.[47]

The Centers for Disease Control and Prevention recommended in 2004 that infants and pregnant women should be vaccinated with the flu shot. Yet, when a pregnant woman is vaccinated with the flu shot, her unborn child receives several hundred times more mercury than US federal agencies claim is safe for adults. Even the vaccine manufacturers who profit from the sale of flu shots state that the vaccine hasn't been adequately tested.

According to Aventis Pasteur, Inc., the makers of Fluzone, a flu vaccine, "Animal reproduction studies have not been conducted with Influenza Virus Vaccine. It is not known whether Influenza Virus Vaccine can cause fetal harm when administered to a pregnant woman or can affect reproduction capacity."

According to Mercola and Klinghardt, in most children the largest source of mercury is that received from immunizations or that transferred to them in utero from their mother." [48]

Dr. Ayoub indicates that the evidence is clear: mercury, particularly from childhood vaccinations, is playing a large role in the incidence of autism. In the article, "Calculate Your Child's Risk of Mercury Poisoning from Vaccines," he states that mercury is "directly linked to the development of autism spectrum disorders and is significantly toxic to the gastrointestinal, immunological, metabolic, and neurobiological systems in children." [49] For more information about autism and a natural approach to its treatment, see chapter 9.

ELIMINATING HEAVY METALS AND MOVING FORWARD

While our environmental, food, supplement, and medical exposure to neurotoxic heavy metals seems overwhelming, in the chapters that follow you'll learn more about what you can do to lessen your exposure to these harmful heavy metals and how to reduce your body's toxic burden of cadmium, aluminum, lead, and mercury using *The Brain Wash* toxic metal elimination program.

chapter
3
The Deadly Neurotoxins

"Two things are infinite: the universe and human stupidity, and I'm not sure about the universe."
~ Albert Einstein

▪ ▪ ▪ ▪ ▪ ▪ ▪

In chapter 3, "The Deadly Neurotoxins," you will learn

- about the growing incidence of brain diseases;
- that exposure to toxic chemicals is increasingly being linked to brain diseases;
- what a "toxic load" and "body burden" are, and why these are important to your brain;
- the high cost of pesticides;
- the link between pesticides and brain and nervous system disorders;
- how to lessen your exposure to pesticides;
- why choosing a better mattress is so important to your brain health;
- how common drugs like hormone replacement therapy, Ritalin, and vaccines affect the brain;
- the high cost of beauty and why you need to avoid products containing fragrance; and
- that fabric softeners and dryer sheets contain many toxic ingredients that can have potentially harmful effects on the brain.

▪ ▪ ▪ ▪ ▪ ▪ ▪

Headlines around the world are reporting two disturbing trends: the incidence of brain disease is growing at an alarming rate; and, increasing levels of industrial chemicals are being found in human bodies.

In 2004, Britain's *The Observer* reported, "The numbers of sufferers of brain diseases, including Alzheimer's, Parkinson's, and motor neuron disease, have soared across the West in less than twenty years."[1] Around the same time, the University of British Columbia released research anticipating that brain disease will be the number one killer of North Americans within only fifteen years.

Montreal's *The Gazette* cited a recent study by Environmental Defence revealing that children as young as ten are showing signs of contamination by toxic chemicals including insecticides and other toxins found in non-stick frying pans, computers, mattresses, and furniture treated with stain repellents. Some of the chemicals found are known causes of neurological problems and developmental disorders in children, among other diseases. The study states that of the chemicals found, thirty-eight are carcinogens, twenty-three are hormone disruptors, twelve are respiratory toxins, thirty-eight are reproductive or developmental toxins, and nineteen are known neurotoxins.

▨ ▨ ▨ ▨ ▨ ▨ ▨

"These are nasty diseases: people are getting more of them and they are starting earlier. We have to look at the environment and ask ourselves what we are doing."[2]
Professor Colin Pritchard, *Journal of Public Health*

▨ ▨ ▨ ▨ ▨ ▨ ▨

According to the article in *The Observer*, a *Journal of Public Health* report examined the incidence of brain diseases in the United Kingdom, United States, Japan, Australia, Canada, France, Germany, Italy, Netherlands, and Spain between 1979 and 1997. The report found that dementias, mainly Alzheimer's-linked dementias, rose sharply in all countries, particularly England and Wales, where there was an alarming increase of more than three hundred percent for men and nearly ninety percent among women.

Scientists ruled out genetic causes because changes to DNA would take hundreds of years to take effect. They concluded by stating the cause "must be the environment."[3]

Researchers believe that chemicals from car pollution, pesticides on crops, and industrial chemicals used on almost every aspect of modern life, from processed food to packaging, electrical goods to sofa covers, are to blame. Alzheimer's was shown to increase in Japanese people when they moved to other countries, making food one of the researchers' major concerns.

So which is the culprit, food or the environment? The two cannot be separated, of course, which leads us to the most challenging problem we face in regard to toxic chemicals: multiple interactions. All of the chemicals that we expose ourselves to co-mingle in our bodies and in our bloodstreams. There are rarely, if ever, any studies done on the multiple interactions of the pollutants to which we are exposed. The researchers in the *Journal of Public Health* report stated that "multiple pollution" is a potential factor for the rapidly rising incidence of these diseases.

Today there are over one hundred studies linking environmental, nutritional, and lifestyle factors to initiating or accelerating brain disease. That's a massive body of evidence by anyone's standards. And, it's something to be concerned about. It's so alarming that the WWF (formerly the World Wildlife Fund) named chemical pollution as one of the two great environmental threats to the world, alongside global warming. In a news report, WWF's toxics program leader, Matthew Wilkinson stated, "We've started seeing changes in fertility rates, the immune system, neurological changes [and] impacts on behaviour."[4]

TOXIC LOAD AND BODY BURDEN

The Mount Sinai School of Medicine in New York and two non-profit groups conducted a study to determine the number of toxic chemicals found in average people. They tested nine volunteers to determine the presence of 210 chemicals commonly found in consumer products and industrial pollutants. Tests on blood and urine found an average of ninety-one industrial compounds, pollutants, and other chemicals in the volunteers, with a total of 167 found across the entire group. Researchers selected people who did not work with chemicals or live in industrial areas. The study demonstrated what is known as "toxic load," or "body burden."

Researchers also noted some troubling findings:

- Children have twice the levels of certain pesticides in their blood than adults;
- Children have higher levels of nicotine than adults;
- Children have higher levels of certain chemicals used in soft plastic toys;
- Adolescents have high levels of phthalates from personal care products;
- Mexican-Americans have three times the levels of the banned pesticide, DDT, in their systems as other Americans.[5]

We all have a toxic load due to a lifetime of exposure to toxins in our environment, water, and food. These toxins accumulate in our body's tissues, particularly in fat stores, as you learned earlier. Because of the high percentage of fat in the brain, it is particularly vulnerable. Airborne toxins present an additional concern since they enter through the nasal passages and can pass directly across the blood-brain barrier into the brain.

THE ENVIRONMENT TODAY

Over four billion pounds of toxic chemicals are released annually into the environment by industry.[6] Currently there are over eighty thousand industrial chemicals in use, and approximately two thousand new chemical compounds are introduced annually.[7] Almost none have been tested for the effects of combined exposures to two or more chemicals. Yet, we are exposed to potentially eighty thousand chemicals combined.

There are many sources of air pollution alone. Some are natural, but most air pollution is human-caused. There are petrochemicals from transportation, such as buses, cars, planes, and transport trucks. Fuel combustion factories, refineries and power plants, as well as industrial manufacturing facilities, spew out toxic chemicals in droves. Waste and waste disposal processes create air pollution. Aerial and land spraying of farms, electromagnetic and electrical emissions, and chemical dumps, all create air pollutants.[8]

Toxic industrial waste is not released solely into the atmosphere; waste is pumped into the ground as well. In 1996, over one billion pounds of chemical emissions were pumped into the air, while an additional 418 million pounds of chemicals were released into the ground.[9] Just four years later, in the year 2000, the amount of atmospheric emissions had doubled to two billion pounds, while almost TEN TIMES the amount of industrial waste, four billion pounds of chemicals, was dumped into the ground.

According to the National Research Council, no toxicity data are available for eighty percent of the chemicals currently in commercial use,[10] while ninety-five percent of chemicals have not been tested for their long-term affects on human health. Virtually no studies test the combined effects of exposure to two or more chemicals on human health. J. Robert Hatherhill, a Stanford University-trained research scientist, indicates, "Many neurotoxic agents combined in low doses may show significant toxicity even though they show little when given alone."[11]

THE HIGH COST OF PESTICIDE USE

More than 1.2 billion pounds of pesticides are used in the United States alone.[12] That equates to three pounds of pesticides and herbicides applied each year for every man, woman, and child in the United States.[13] Approximately ten percent of these products are applied to lawns and gardens, and the remainder are used in industrial, agricultural, and commercial applications, all of which contributes extensively to the contamination of the environment, our bodies, and our children's bodies.

The World Health Organization estimates that one-half of the ground and well water in the United States is contaminated with pesticides.[14] Pesticides travel in the air and are carried by wind to destinations miles away from the application site. Pesticides are washed into our streams, lakes, rivers, and underground aquifers that supply our drinking and bathing water, and these poisons are making their way into our bodies. The herbicide 2, 4-D, was found in fifty percent of semen samples taken from Canadian men.[15] That's a scary proposition when one considers that semen carries the genetic material of a possible fetus or child.

Another pesticide, chlorpyrifos (CPF), was found in eighty-two percent of urine samples from a broad range of Americans aged twenty to fifty-nine. These are just two examples of the 891 pesticides and herbicides registered with the Environmental Protection Agency at the time of writing of this book.

A new study on the ill-effects of pesticides pops up faster than you can say "DDT." The University of Rochester School of Medicine and Dentistry conducted a study of a common herbicide, paraquat, and a common fungicide, maneb. Mice that were subjected to these chemicals developed the same pattern of brain damage seen in Parkinson's disease. Pesticides and herbicides are increasingly linked to other brain and neurological disorders, as well as heart, lung, kidney, and adrenal gland diseases. Richard Mesquita describes the effects of pesticides and herbicides in his article, "Pesticide and Herbicide Contamination":

> The intent of pesticide or herbicide applications is to kill various pests or weeds they come in contact with. And most of these toxins do that job very well. But that also means when we're exposed to them, they try to do the same thing to us. Yet since we are larger and are made a little differently, it seems they only do part of the job. Hence, we **don't die immediately**, but instead **live debilitated lives**.[16]

According to Doris J. Rapp, MD, author of *Our Toxic World: A Wake Up Call*, pesticides, and other chemicals found in human tissue, have been found to alter *the brain and nervous system causing headaches, difficulty thinking or remembering, inexplicable emotional ups and downs, inconsolable depression, irritability, moodiness, aggression, hyperactivity or extreme fatigue...[pesticides also affect] the muscular system causing twitches, tics, muscle pains or weakness, in time possibly leading to fibromyalgia, multiple sclerosis, amyotrophic lateral sclerosis or Parkinson's disease.*[17]

Dr. Rapp also cites research in the same book linking pesticide exposure to multiple sclerosis.[18]

Because the use of pesticides is so prevalent, every child conceived today in the Northern Hemisphere will be exposed to pesticides in the womb or within the first year after birth.[19] Remember my earlier discussion about the first few years of brain development? Exposure to toxins during critical times causes a child to be much more vulnerable to brain diseases during childhood or later in adulthood. Yet, scientists can't say for sure what those critical times in development are.

Even schoolyards pose a threat to children. Schools spray herbicides, insecticides, fungicides, pesticides, rodent baits, disinfectants, wood preservatives, soil sterilants, and other chemicals on playground areas to control pests and other problems. While some schools set their own standards, little if any regulations exist to determine what substances are used around school-aged children, who are more vulnerable to the effects of these chemicals. Some US senators have publicly expressed their concern and have even stated that most workplaces have far stricter standards than do schools. Schools have a responsibility to children to help them develop their minds, not unknowingly subject them to neurotoxins during their most vulnerable years.

CPF, also known as Dursban, and a known nervous system poison,[20] is used on many schoolyards and playgrounds. Diazinon, also frequently used on lawns, can trigger many health problems and is also a nervous system poison.[21] According to the National Coalition Against the Misuse of Pesticides, studies link pesticide use to increased rates of many diseases among children, including brain cancer.[22] This must be addressed. The best way to ensure a child's healthy brain development is to minimize toxic exposures.

The National Environmental Trust, Physicians for Social Responsibility, and the Learning Disabilities Association released a joint report in 2000 outlining that US industry releases annually about twenty-four billion pounds of toxic substances believed to cause developmental and neurological problems in children. That amount could fill a string of railroad cars from New York City to Albuquerque, New Mexico, and the report critiqued the government for its lack of emissions standards for these toxic chemicals.[23] Years later, virtually nothing has been done to stop the continual onslaught of industrial chemicals with neurotoxic effects from polluting the environment.

PESTICIDES IN AGRICULTURE

Our greatest exposure to pesticides is through their use in agriculture, although household, lawn, and golf course use also results in sizable quantities of pesticides finding their way into our air, water, and food.

Organophosphates are the most widely used type of pesticides. At least forty different types are in use in homes, gardens, agriculture, and veterinary practice. Organophosphates were originally developed by Nazi chemists during World War II as a chemical weapon nerve agent. Once the war was over, industry found a new use for these nerve agents, in the form of pesticides for lawn "care." The US Department of Defense (DOD) published a 1.5 million dollar study in the journal *Nature Genetics* connecting neurological disorders like attention deficit and hyperactivity disorder (ADHD) and Parkinson's disease with organophosphates. In the study researchers discovered that organophosphates inhibited the activity of a particular gene (neuropathy target esterase), whose function is to let the brain control body movement. The study was conducted to learn more about using organophosphates in chemical weaponry.[24]

Any pesticides used in agriculture find their way directly into our bodies through the food we consume. An apple a day might have kept the doctor away prior to the industrialization of food growing and preparation. But, according to research compiled by the United States Drug Administration (USDA) today's apple contains residue of eleven different neurotoxins—azinphos, methyl chloripyrifos, diazinon, dimethoate, ethion, omthoate, parathion, parathion methyl, phosalone, and phosmet—and the USDA was testing for only one category of chemicals known as organophosphate insecticides. That doesn't sound too appetizing does it? The average apple is sprayed with pesticides seventeen times before it is harvested.[25]

Even so-called "banned" pesticides are showing up in human tissue samples. Many of these chemicals have long-lasting environmental effects. Canadian and North American authorities are often quick to cite that some types of pesticides are banned for use, but they readily allow the legal import of fruits, vegetables, grains, and other products sprayed with these banned pesticides. A substance isn't banned if it can be imported.

*Pesticides Linked with Brain and Nervous System Disorders[26]

Pesticides	Use	Linked To
DDT (banned in Canada and the United States but still found on imported products)	Used against a wide variety of insects	Polyneuritis
Endosulfan	Broad spectrum insecticide	Genetic mutation
Dieldrin	Used against many ticks and lice, as well as to protect fabrics against moths, beetles.	Parkinson's disease Alzheimer's disease
Chlordane	Used in soil against grubs and termites	Brain cancer
Lindane	Used against soil and grain pests	Polyneuritis
Fenthion	Insecticide	Genetic mutation
Phorate	Used against aphids and fruit flies, and to kill worms in potato crops	Neurological and neuromuscular effects
Malathion	Wide use against aphids, mites, and other pests	Genetic mutation Delayed neurotoxin Behavioural effects Abnormal brain waves
Monocrotofos	Broad spectrum insecticide used to control pests on crops like cotton, rice, soybeans, corn, coffee, citrus, and potatoes	Delayed neuropathy
Dimethoate	Used on agriculture and horticultural crops, particularly against spider mites	Genetic mutation

Continued

Pesticides	Use	Linked To
Chlorpyrifos	Broad spectrum insecticide	Neuro-behavioural effects like headaches, blurred vision, unusual fatigue or muscle weakness, problems with memory, concentration, depression, and irritability
Quinalphos	Broad spectrum insecticide	Blocks healthy nerve impulses
Triazophos	Used primarily on cereal grains, corn, carrots, and potatoes	Blocks healthy nerve impulses
Ethion	Used against chewing insects	Genetic mutation
Acephate	Used against chewing insects	Genetic mutation
Permethrin	Contact insecticide, used against pests of cotton, fruit, and vegetable crops	Neurotoxic dangers to fetuses
Carbaryl	Broad spectrum insecticide, used on fruit, vegetable, and cotton crops	Nervous system damage Brain cancer
Carbofuran	Broad spectrum insecticide, used in soil	Blocks healthy nerve impulses Impaired nervous system function
Methomyl	Soil insecticide, used primarily against aphids	Blocks healthy nerve impulses Weakness and muscle aches
Butachlor	Used against grasses and broad-leafed weeds	Reduced brain size Brain lesions
Paraquat	Used against grasses	Parkinson's disease Alzheimer's disease
Catan	Fungicide used on foliage, seed, and soil	Genetic mutation

Continued

*NOTE: Many of these pesticides have been linked to a long list of other symptoms and diseases. I've restricted the chart to include brain and nervous system diseases, and genetic mutation.

Of course, every now and then a study is unveiled that indicates pesticides are not harmful and are not linked to disease. Most of these studies do not consider long-term exposure, the cumulative effects of pesticides and other chemicals our bodies are exposed to throughout our lifetimes, interactions between multiple chemicals, the effects on people who have compromised immune systems, and of course, children whose bodies are developing. Many of these studies are also funded by the very industry that has a vested interest in keeping pesticides on store shelves and sprayed on lawns. Sometimes this funding is overt, but often it is provided by a so-called "independent research institute" that derives its funding from corporate players in the chemical industry.

Parkinson's Disease Linked to Pesticide Use

The British government's Advisory Committee on Pesticides ordered a review of all studies linking pesticides to Parkinson's disease. Because numerous studies have shown that people living in rural areas, where exposure to pesticides is more likely, are at a higher risk of developing Parkinson's disease, scientists have been reviewing the studies to determine if a specific pesticide, or class of pesticides, is linked to Parkinson's. These scientists believe that exposure to certain pesticides may trigger Parkinson's by stopping brain cells from producing adequate amounts of a brain messenger hormone called dopamine.[27]

Lorene Nelson, PhD, a neuroepidemiologist at Stanford University School of Medicine, and her colleagues conducted a study of 496 people diagnosed with Parkinson's disease and 541 people without the disease, to determine lifetime insecticide, herbicide, and fungicide use, exposure, and frequency. They determined that people who had the highest exposure to pesticides were twice as likely to develop Parkinson's disease than people not exposed to the chemicals. Past exposure to herbicides was also associated with the disease. Researchers suspect that damage to nerve cells in the *substantia nigra* part of the brain as a result of exposure to chemicals that accumulate in this area, may cause movement difficulties characteristic of Parkinson's disease. Researchers stressed that pesticide use is a public health issue.[28]

There is further evidence to support the growing body of research that Parkinson's disease is linked to environmental factors, especially pesticides. Researchers found that injection of two pesticides, the herbicide paraquat and fungicide maneb, resulted in an immediate reduction in the motor activity of mice. Analysis of the mice's brains revealed extensive damage to the nigrostriatal system, which is the same area of the brain affected in humans with Parkinson's disease. The damage did not occur when either pesticide was injected on its own. Paraquat is similar to another chemical, MPTP, which is known to produce Parkinson's. The researchers believe that maneb either heightens the toxicity of paraquat or enables it to cross the blood-brain barrier.[29]

Another study revealed that several pesticides can cause cellular damage that resembles Parkinson's disease. Previously, research linked the pesticide rotenone with symptoms and features like Parkinson's disease seen in rats. Newer research links additional pesticides to the same cellular damage. Dr. Todd B. Sherer and his colleagues at Emory University in Atlanta discovered that pyridaben and fenpyroximate caused similar damage to that caused by rotenone. Pyridaben proved even more toxic, however.[30]

Futuristic Pesticides: A Horror Show

The future of agriculture and our food supply could harbour something even more worrisome than pesticides over the coming years. Scientists are testing out a new delivery method for pesticides, which they refer to as "ghost bugs." Researchers take empty shells of bacteria, fill them with pesticides, and infect the bacterial cells with a virus, then unleash these mutants onto plants.

In preliminary research in which these ghosts were filled with a fungicide called "tebuconazole," and compared to simply spraying the fungicide directly onto barley and wheat, researchers found the ghost bugs' pesticide activity was higher. In other studies, tebuconazole has been linked to learning disorders in rats. What are the possible human effects of ingesting these virus-infected bacteria filled with toxic chemicals? That's still to be determined. Organic produce is sounding better every day.

■ ■ ■ ■ ■ ■ ■

Lessen Your Exposure to Pesticides!
There are simple ways to lessen your exposure to pesticides:

- Stop using pesticides, herbicides, and insecticides in your home, on your lawn, or on any plants;
- Eat organic food as much as possible;
- Determine if your water is free of any pesticides, herbicides, or other toxins, and obtain an appropriate water treatment system if necessary.

You cannot tell if your water is safe simply by how it smells, looks, or tastes. Some contaminants are harmful even in parts per billion. Installing a water filtration system to purify your drinking water may be inadequate. Your body absorbs many chemicals through your skin and through steam inhalation during showers and baths. Consider a whole home water purification system which will reduce or eliminate organophosphates and other chemicals in all water.

■ ■ ■ ■ ■ ■ ■

SMOKE GETS IN YOUR EYES... AND FIRE RETARDANTS GET IN YOUR BRAIN

Pesticides are not the only neurotoxic industrial chemicals to be wary of. Fire retardants are finding their way into the environment through our food supply, our water and air, and in many consumer goods like furniture and mattresses. What's more, fire retardants are showing up in human tissue samples from all around the globe. Even polar bears in the Arctic, with seemingly no exposure to these toxic substances, are contaminated.

The ABCs of PBDEs

A group of commonly used fire retardants, called polybrominated dithenyl ethers (PBDEs), can harm neurological development and function in babies and young children, just like mercury and PCBs. These toxic chemicals are added to common household and workplace items like computers, electronics, televisions, upholstered furniture, mattresses, carpets, stereos, seat cushions, clothing, and synthetic fabrics.[31]

Ironically, fire retardants have been used as a "safety precaution" when added to consumer products. These retardants were tested in the 1980s and were found to be safe, but more sophisticated and recent testing for hormone-like effects has found them to be highly toxic.

In recent research, fire retardants demonstrated an ability to mimic thyroid hormones, and it is believed that they follow a hormonal route, until they play havoc on the brain, causing such effects as hyperactivity and impaired learning.[32] According to an article in Canada's *The Globe and Mail* newspaper, "the traditional mantra of toxicologists has been that the dose makes the poison," which, translated, means that the dose of a chemical substance has to be large to have an effect. States the author of the article, Martin Mittelstaedt, "The amounts used…are the lowest seen to produce effects, are approaching levels seen in some people in North America, and were thousands of times smaller than the amounts found to kill test animals." The article also cited a biologist at the University of Massachusetts, Dr. Thomas Zoeller, who is studying fire retardants for the US Environmental Protection Agency. He indicated that the behavioural effects persisted as the rodents aged, implying that the damage from the chemicals was permanent. He stated, "You either prevent these [effects] or you cope with them."

Another study found that sometimes the dose of the chemical is less important than the point in an animal's life when the animal is exposed. Mice aged four- and ten-days old were given traces of fire retardants and subsequently exhibited behavioural abnormalities; but, the same dose given to nineteen-day old mice caused no change compared to the control animals. "Scientists theorize that the flame retardants had their effect by interfering with hormones during the period of rapid brain growth in the rodents in the first two weeks of life. In humans, this brain growth spurt lasts from the final part of pregnancy through the first two years of life."[33] The amount of flame retardant that found its way into brain tissue was only ten parts per trillion, or the equivalent of ten grains of salt in an Olympic-size swimming pool, yet its effects were damaging and permanent.

Studies are finding fire retardants in more than just commercial and household items, which concerns researchers. A study published in *Environmental Science & Technology*, a peer-reviewed journal of the American Chemical Society, found higher levels of fire retardants in American foods than in similar foods from other countries. PBDEs contaminated all tested food that contained animal fats, with the highest levels found in fish, then meat, followed by dairy products. [34]

In the report, Dr. Schecter states, "although these findings are preliminary, they suggest that food is a major route of intake for PBDEs."[35] As I mentioned earlier, most toxins, PBDEs included, are fat-soluble and are stored in fat. In this case, PBDEs are stored in the seafood and animals that make up part of our food supply. Then the chemicals find their way into fatty stores in the body, and can possibly travel across the blood-brain barrier into the brain.

Once ingested, PBDEs make their way through the body, including into women's breast milk. In a study of the breast milk of women in Dallas and Austin, scientists found the highest levels in the world to date.[36] They believe this is due to the high concentrations of PBDEs found in the foods the women are eating. A separate study indicated that North American women currently have PBDE levels that are twenty to forty times higher than European women. The amount of PBDEs in Canadian women's breast milk is second only to American women. But the news gets worse. Additional research reveals that PBDE levels in women's breast milk are doubling every four to five years.

Some European Union countries have taken action against PBDEs. Sweden has not allowed PBDE use for many years and their strong stance is paying off. The levels in breast milk are falling. In 2004, the

European Union passed legislation banning the manufacture and use of PBDEs. In a report prepared by the Labour Environmental Alliance Society in Canada, leading PBDE researcher Ake Bergman states, "We already know more about PBDEs than we knew about PCBs when we banned them in the 1970s. It's really time to act."[37]

The federal government in Canada has known about the toxic nature of fire retardants since as early as 2004. After screening them as part of the Canadian Environmental Protection Act, Environment Canada concluded, "All PBDEs have the potential to transform to other compounds of concern. Based on this evidence, it is concluded that PBDEs [of many types]… may have an immediate or long-term harmful effect on the environment or its biological diversity and are considered to be 'toxic'…"

At the time of writing of this book, the Canadian federal government plans to add both PBDEs and perfluorooctane sulfonate to its list of toxic substances, which would be one of the most aggressive stances on these fire retardants in the world. It's an action I hope to see become a reality by the time this book is released. The Canadian government is also planning tight controls on other fire retardants. This would be an important decision since regulators have determined that about four thousand chemicals that have been used for decades in Canada pose a potential threat to human health and the environment. These four thousand chemicals were culled from a list of twenty-three thousand industrial chemicals that were grandfathered through the regulations prior to Canada initiating pollution legislation.

Because fire retardants are in such widespread use, it can be difficult to avoid them, but it is possible to lessen your exposure. The best place to start is with your mattress.

To Sleep Perchance to Dream?

Maybe Hamlet needed a flame-retardant-free mattress when he uttered these words of torment. Most commercially-purchased mattresses are sprayed with flame retardants, among other things. But, it is possible to obtain a mattress that's free of these toxic substances. They are pricier than the typical mattress, but considering that we spend eight hours a night breathing in any off-gassing chemicals, the expense is well worth the health benefits.

I've found a couple of options, depending on health needs and preferences. The main ones are organic cotton (make sure it is one hundred percent organic) or one hundred percent natural latex. Some manufacturers of organic beds also manufacture organic pillows. Natural latex is harvested sustainably from the rainforest, ensuring that the trees are left intact. Be sure that the mattress you choose is free from all synthetic chemicals like fire retardants. One hundred percent organic cotton mattresses are also free of the bleaches, pesticides, dyes, resins, formaldehyde, and other chemicals that are found in traditional cotton mattresses.

For more information about these products and where you can purchase them, consult the resource section at the back of this book.

THE PITFALLS OF PILL-POPPING

We've covered many of the environmental sources for toxins that are impairing our brain's ability to function, including toxic waste and pollution, multiple chemical interaction, pesticides, and fire retardants, all of which are making their way into our systems through the air we breathe and the foods we eat. Now, there are several other culprits that are easily avoided once you know what to look out for. Let's take a look at some of the most common and harmful habits we've acquired as a society, and learn how to avoid these additional chemicals altogether.

Ritalin May Cause Brain Damage

While ADD and ADHD are very much on the rise, as are brain health problems globally, experts believe that there are many, many cases of misdiagnosis. If you believe your child may be suffering from ADD, I encourage you to turn to chapter 9 to learn about the defining characteristics of these diseases to ensure you have a credible diagnosis of this serious disorder (and not just an active, distracted, normal kid going through a growth spurt, for example!), and to carefully follow *The*

Brain Wash Plan for both yourself and your children. The drugs offered to combat ADD and ADHD have unfortunately been shown time and time again to cause further damage to the brain. For example, childhood Ritalin use is linked to adult depression and anxiety. American scientists believe that Ritalin alters the brain's chemical composition so that it has a lasting effect on mental health. Because a child's brain is growing and developing, the result of Ritalin use could cause irreversible brain damage.[38] British doctors dispensed 254, 000 Ritalin prescriptions in 2002 alone. According to some estimates, one in twenty children is believed to have ADHD, which makes them hyperactive and unfocused. However, other experts observe that the diagnosis is frequently made without the many defining characteristics of ADHD, and without any testing.

I am concerned with the over-prescription of Ritalin, and many parents' attempt to find a quick fix for their children's behavioural problems. Weigh the benefits and risks of Ritalin use carefully.

Vaccines

According to an article entitled, "The Age of Autism: A pretty big secret" by Dan Olmsted, there may be a link between autism and vaccination. He refers to The Homefirst Health Services in Chicago. According to the medical director, Dr. Mayer Eisenstein, Homefirst has delivered more than fifteen thousand babies and cared for thirty to thirty-five thousand children since the health centre's inception in 1973. During that time, he claims that the facility has not seen a single case of autism in thousands of children who have never been vaccinated.[39]

The few autistic children Homefirst sees were vaccinated prior to becoming patients. According to the article, Dr. Eisenstein feels that they have enough samples to be statistically relevant. Eisenstein is the author of the book *Don't Vaccinate Before You Educate!* He is wary of the Centers for Disease Control's vaccination policy from the 1990s that added several new immunizations to the schedule, including immunizing against hepatitis B as early as the date of birth.

Pediatrician Dr. Jeff Bradstreet also cited in the Homefirst article, stated there is virtually no autism in home-schooling families who decline to vaccinate for religious reasons.

Health authorities, which seem to be the biggest vaccine pushers, claim there is no link between autism and vaccines. And a recent study suggested they were right. The study's authors even went as far as to state their independence from any vaccine manufacturers. Yet, the study was funded by a non-profit group whose members include numerous big name pharmaceutical companies. Independent, huh?

In 2005, the global vaccine market was estimated at 5.8 billion dollars,[40] small by pharmaceutical standards but big bucks by just about everyone else's. Plus, IMS Health, a company that tracks the pharmaceutical industry's sales, indicates vaccine sales are estimated to increase by twenty percent per year over the next five years.[41]

There is also anecdotal evidence that the Amish, who are not vaccinated for religious reasons, are virtually untouched by autism.

The research is still out on the effect of vaccines on the brain, but it is important to consider the potential consequences prior to blindly vaccinating a child. And doctors need to stop bullying parents into making any decisions about vaccinations. Too many doctors cite morals and ethics as a means to push parents into vaccinating children. While there is plenty of bullying in the health industry, there's no room for bullying when it comes to health.

THE HIGH COST OF BEAUTY

The use of common soaps, shampoos, hairspray, and deodorants can have a negative impact on your brain and nervous system health. Most popular brands of cosmetics are loaded with artificial colours, synthetic fragrances, petroleum products, emulsifiers, preservatives, and solvents. Over 850 toxic chemicals are available for use in makeup. Some of these ingredients are proven carcinogens—they are linked to causing cancer. Others have damaging effects on the nervous system. Still others are mutagens, which means they are products that can cause changes to the information in your body's cellular genetic material and potentially lead to genetic disease.

Sodium lauryl sulphate, one of the synthetic substances used in shampoos and soaps for its foaming properties, causes many allergic reactions. It is also a known mutagen.

Stearalkonium chloride is another toxic chemical used in many hair conditioners and moisturizers. Originally developed by the fabric industry as a fabric softener, this toxic ingredient found its way into skin and hair products because it is much less expensive than proteins and natural ingredients. Unfortunately, this toxin also causes many allergic reactions.

A "FRAGRANCE" BY ANY OTHER NAME...

An article that appeared in *The Townsend Letter for Doctors and Patients* indicates that "perfumes contain neurotoxins, which have a causal link to central nervous system disorders, headaches, confusion, dizziness, short-term memory loss, anxiety, depression, disorientation, and mood swings."[42] The author of the article explains that fragrance inhalation through the nose goes directly to the brain where it can have neurological effects.

That perfume, cologne, laundry detergent, and other personal "care" product that you think makes you smell attractive is more likely damaging your health and having negative implications for your brain and moods.

Perfumes contain neurotoxins that have been linked as causes for a variety of nervous system disorders, including short-term memory loss and depression. As early as the 1970s, a series of animal studies found that a synthetic fragrance ingredient called musk tetralin (AETT) was causing significant brain and spinal cord damage, but it continued to be allowed in consumer products for many years before the cosmetics industry stopped using it.[43] Today there are hundreds of ingredients still in use in everyday perfumes, colognes, hairsprays, and air "fresheners" that research has proven to be toxic.

Below, you'll find a chart that indicates some of the most common fragrance ingredients and their toxic effects. Pick up your shampoo bottle and find out what's really being massaged onto your scalp every morning! If you don't see a list of ingredients, the manufacturer may have something to hide.

Comon Fragrance Ingredients

Name of Ingredients	Found In	Toxic Effects
Acetaldehyde	Perfume, dyes, packaged or prepared food, and fish preservatives	Studies of animals show that acetaldehyde crosses the placenta to the fetus Probable human carcinogen
Acetone	Cologne, diswashing detergent, nail polish remover, and cosmetics	Central nervous system effects such as dizziness, nausea, drowsiness, loss of coordination, tremors, and comas
Acetonitrile	Perfume, dyes, and pharmaceutical drugs	Central nervous system effects such as weakness, headaches, tremors, numbness, convulsions, and death
Benzyl Alcohol	Perfume, cologne, shampoo, air fresheners, laundry bleach, detergent, fabric softener, deodorants, soap, nail polish remover, cosmetics, pharmaceutical drugs, and ointments	Central nervous system effects such as dizziness, headahces, fatigue, and weakness
Benzyl Chloride	Perfume, dyes, pharmaceutical drugs, and prepared or packaged food * Formerly used as an irritant gas in chemical warfare	Central nervous system effects include dizziness, headaches, and fatigue A suspected animal carcinogen
Dimenthyl Sulphate	Perfume, dyes, and pharmaceutical drugs * Formerly used as an irritant gas in chemical warfare	Probable human carcinogen Severe exposure can cause central nervous system damage, convulsions, delirium, paralysis, comas, and death

Continued

Name of Ingredients	Found In	Toxic Effects
Ethanol	Perfume, hairspray, shampoo, air "fresheners," nail polish, nail polish remover, laundry detergent, shaving cream, and dishwashing detergent	Central nervous system effects include fatigue and tremors
Linalool	Perfume, cologne, air "fresheners," aftershave, shaving cream, soap, hand lotion, fabric softnerer, laundry detergent, and dishwashing liquid	Central nervous system effects include confusion, depression, and dizziness
Methylene Chloride (dichloromethane)	Shampoo, cologne, paint, and varnish remover * Banned by the US FDA in 1988 but based on a 1991 EPA Report on Fragrances it was still found in fragranced products.	Carcinogenic. Central nervous system effects include headaches, numbness, irritability, fatigue, and confusion Linked with central nervous system damage Severe exposure can cause loss of consciousness and death
Musk Ambrette	Perfume	Central nervous system effects include damage and muscle weakness in laboratory animals

Continued

Name of Ingredients	Found In	Toxic Effects
Musk Tetralin (AETT)	Perfume, aftershave lotions, colognes, creams, and as a "masking agent" in unscented products * Voluntarily banned by some companies in the fragrance industry as of 1977, but not legally banned. There is no guarantee it is not being used now.	Central nervous system effects include irritablilty, degeneration of brain neurons, and changes in the spinal cord of laboratory animals.
Styrene Oxide	Perfume and cosmetics	Central nervous system effects include depression in animals
a-Terpineol	Perfume, cologne, fabric softner, air "freshners," soap, hairspray, laundry detergent and bleach, and aftershave	Effects include headaches, depression, and central nervous system damage
Toluene (methyl benzene)	Perfume, soap, cosmetics, nail polish removers, detergents, dyes, aerosol spray paints, paint removers, spot removers, gasoline, antifreeze, and explosives * Toluene was detected in every fragrance sample collected by the US EPA in their 1991 report	Central nervous system damage Other central nervous system effects include dizziness, tremors, numbness, headaches, confusion, unconsciousness, memory loss, loss of muscle control, and brain damage, and problems with speech, hearing, and vision

Adapted from S. Moser. "Fragrance Chemicals as Toxic Substances." Citizens for a Safe Learning Environment. http://www.chebucto.ns.ca/Education/CASLE.

Even items that are labelled "fragrance-free" or "unscented" may still contain fragrances thanks to lax laws in Canada and the United States. Companies simply state that their fragrance formulations are "trade secrets" and they are not required to disclose the product's contents to anyone. By these standards, a company's intellectual *property* is seen as more valuable than an individual's right to his or her intellectual *capacity* and the health of the organ from which it stems—the brain.

SOFTNESS OVER SAFETY

One of the most toxic things we do on a regular basis is to use fabric softener or throw a dryer sheet in our laundry. Sounds crazy, I know, but it is true. Fabric softeners and dryer sheets should be banned from public use: they are incredibly full of toxic chemicals that are known to damage the brain and nervous system. Following is a chart of the main ingredients found in most commercial fabric softeners and dryer sheets. Keep in mind, these are just the main ingredients.

Main Ingredients Found in Fabric Softeners and Dryer Sheets

Chemical Ingredient	Known Central Nervous System Effects
Alpha-Terpineol	Causes central nervous system disorders Can also cause loss of muscular coordination, central nervous system depression, and headache
Benzyl Alcohol	Causes central nervous system disorders, headaches, nausea, vomiting, dizziness, central nervous system depression, and, in severe cases, death
Camphor	On the US EPA's Hazardous Waste list Central nervous system stimulant, causes dizziness, confusion, nausea, twitching muscles, and convulsions
Chloroform	On the EPA's Hazardous Waste list Neuotoxic and carcinogenic
Ethyl Acetate	On the EPA's Hazardous Waste list Narcotic May cause headaches and narcosis (stupor)
Linalool	Causes Central nervous system disorders. Narcotic In studies of animals, it caused ataxic gait (loss of muscular coordination), reduced spontaneous motor activity, and depression
Pentane	Causes headaches, nausea, vomiting, dizziness, drowsiness, and loss of consciousness Repeated inhalation of vapours causes central nervous system depression

Adapted from "Material Safety Data Sheets." MSDS. http://www.mdsdonline.com.

SURVIVING THE NEUROTOXINS

In 2004, NewScientist.com aptly described the effects of pollutants in animals: "hyperactive fish, stupid frogs, fearless mice, and seagulls that fall over. It sounds like a weird animal circus but this is no freak show. Animals around the world are increasingly behaving in bizarre ways, and the cause is environmental pollution." For decades, biologists have known that PCBs, heavy metals, and other toxic pollutants can alter the behaviour of wild animals. Two new studies have independently shown that these chemicals alter learning, activity levels, and balance, among other things.

Too often we isolate ourselves from the animal kingdom in favour of the absurd notion that we are somehow invulnerable to the effects of increasingly toxic air, water, and food. Research is clearly showing that humans are suffering the brain and neurological effects of pollution.

Knowing where these harmful neurotoxins hide is the first step in learning how to lessen and prevent their effects. It is also essential to detoxify to prevent the build-up of neurotoxins in our tissues or brain. Keep reading to learn how you can combat neurotoxins using proven foods, natural medicines, and holistic therapies.

c h a p t e r
4

Foods, Pseudo-Foods, and Chemicals in Disguise

"To my mind, one of the greatest offences against a man is to deprive him of the normal supply of nourishment during infancy. It gives a bad start. He is shorn of his natural rights... The present abundance of nursing bottles and infants' foods in the drug stores is evidence of degeneration... Shall our children be sacrificed?"

~ Ephraim Cutter, MD

▨ ▨ ▨ ▨ ▨ ▨ ▨

In chapter 4, "Foods, Pseudo-Foods and Chemicals in Disguise," you will learn

- how children are being deprived of essential nutrients to grow healthy brains;
- how parents are unknowingly bombarding children with toxins known to disrupt healthy brain development;
- why breastfeeding an infant is essential to his or her brain health for life;
- how healthy fats build superior brain health and mental capacity;
- the many places harmful food additives like MSG lurk, and why you need to avoid them;
- why sugar and artificial sweeteners are not the healthy stuff you might believe them to be;
- why you need to stop eating brain-destructive hydrogenated and trans fats and the foods in which they are found;
- how insidious food additives accumulate in your diet, and the harmful effects of eating them; and
- the most common neurotoxic foods to avoid.

▨ ▨ ▨ ▨ ▨ ▨ ▨

Now that you have an understanding of the environmental toxins our amazing bodies deal with on a regular basis, this chapter will introduce you to the final hiding place for dangerous chemicals that wreak havoc on our powerful brains: food. It is a hiding place few people look, and one that is host to thousands of different toxic substances.

Your brain requires oxygen and all the essential amino acids in suitable proportions to create adequate neurotransmitters that ensure proper brain cell communication, and therefore proper bodily functioning. The body needs healthy carbohydrates to provide fuel for the brain. In addition, your brain requires adequate amounts of healthy fats to create a stable, protective membrane around individual brain cells and surrounding the brain itself. It requires adequate vitamins and minerals to create healthy brain cells that function properly and will not be slated for a premature death. It needs adequate water (not coffee, tea, or cola) to ensure the proper fluid balance in the brain.

So what happens when, instead of all the essential nutrients needed for brain health, the brain receives suboptimal nutrients, rancid or chemically-altered fats, incorrect amino acid balance thanks to food processing, insufficient water, and excessive amounts of sugar, synthetic sweeteners, artificial colours, and other food additives? Let's find out.

PESTICIDES AND ADDITIVES FOR OUR BABIES?

According to research by the Environmental Working Group (EWG), a watchdog environmental organization, ninety percent of children under the age of five are exposed to neurotoxins in baby food. The EWG also found that commercial baby food provides unsafe levels of a particular type of pesticide.[1] Their research of some popular brands of baby food found neurotoxins in many familiar foods.

Neurotoxins and Baby Food

- Pear purée: five known neurotoxic pesticides.
- Peach purée: four neurotoxic or carcinogenic pesticides.
- Applesauce purée: four neurotoxic pesticides.

- Plum purée: three carcinogenic or neurotoxic pesticides.
- Green bean purée: three neurotoxic pesticides.[2]

If toxic pesticide residues in baby food aren't enough, consider that manufacturers of baby food routinely add synthetic flavour-enhancers and other additives to baby food that are harmful. And their favourite additive? MSG.

MSG: THE LITTLE ADDITIVE THAT COULD... DAMAGE YOUR BRAIN

Monosodium glutamate, better known as MSG, is a pervasive chemical added to foods to enhance flavour. There is a growing body of research that proves this commonly used additive is a potent neurotoxin.

Research suggests that over-activity of a brain messenger called glutamate, a protein precursor that causes excitation of certain brain cells and neurons, may lead to brain cell death and Parkinson's progression.[3] Monosodium glutamate has excitotoxic properties, which means that MSG can over-excite brain cells until they die.

Most people react within forty-eight hours of ingesting (even a small amount) of MSG, making it somewhat difficult to trace back to the originating food item. Symptoms can include: headaches, hives, mouth eruptions, swelling of mucous membranes (in the oral, gastrointestinal, or reproductive tract), runny nose, insomnia, seizures, mood swings, panic attacks, diarrhea, heart palpitations and other cardiac irregularities, nausea, numbness, burning, tingling, chest pain, asthma attacks, and migraines—symptoms most people believe are allergic reactions.

These symptoms are NOT allergic reactions, the symptoms are the result of ingesting a substance that induces nervous system changes and possible nerve damage. According to Dr. Patricia Fitzgerald, "Ingesting MSG over the years has also been linked with Parkinson's and Alzheimer's."[4]

Would you believe commercial baby food manufacturers add MSG to baby food? True. And one of the worst culprits for hidden MSG is infant formula. Most popular brands of infant formula contain MSG in one form or another. MSG is capable of causing permanent damage to an adult nervous system, but is especially toxic to a growing child. Call the manufacturers and they'll tell you that baby food doesn't contain this potent neurotoxin. But, what they won't tell you is that they add other ingredients that make up the harmful constituents of MSG, namely various forms of glutamate.

Most people are aware that MSG is frequently found in Chinese food, but it masquerades under different names in many food ingredients, so don't be surprised if you don't see it labelled as MSG on ingredient lists. Manufacturers who choose to include MSG under a different name, as its component parts or as derivatives of this harmful ingredient, are tricking unsuspecting consumers who rely on their products. Essentially, only the name differs, not the ingredient's capacity to cause brain damage. And MSG by any other name would still be as harmful. This nervous system toxin is also contained in many other food additives.

Sources of MSG

- Autolyzed yeast
- Calcium caseinate
- Gelatin
- Glutamate
- Glutamic acid
- Hydrolyzed protein
- Hydrolyzed soy protein
- Hydrolyzed vegetable protein
- Monopotassium glutamate
- Sodium caseinate
- Yeast extract
- Yeast food
- Yeast nutrient[5]

But, MSG is not only found in baby food. If you're eating in fast food restaurants, "family" restaurants, or purchasing packaged or prepared foods, you're most likely ingesting MSG on a regular basis. This dangerous additive can be found in flavours added to many foods and often labelled as "natural flavour," "natural beef or chicken flavouring," or "natural flavouring." One of the most common places you'll find MSG lurking is in soup, since bouillon, broth, and stock frequently contains MSG.

Because the additive has so many guises, most restaurateurs may believe their food is devoid of MSG, and may advertise it as such, when in reality it may be loaded with the harmful additive. Chefs and restaurateurs, like other members of the public, simply can't keep up with the many names of MSG. You're less likely to find MSG hidden in your food at higher-quality restaurants serving only fresh food, cooked from scratch, without bottled sauces and seasonings.

But, while MSG is insidious in prepared or fast foods, foods are not the only place you're exposed to it. You'll probably be surprised to learn that MSG is found in vaccines as a "stabilizer." The chickenpox vaccine by Merck & Co., Inc. (Merck) is a primary example. Merck's Measles, Mumps, and Rubella vaccine also contains this harmful neurotoxin.

Introduced by the food industry fifty years ago, MSG has been added in larger and larger doses to prepackaged foods, soups, snacks, and fast foods. Think your "health foods" are unspoiled by MSG? Think again. Start reading labels looking for the many guises of MSG. If you find any of the terms listed above, you can bet it's a derivative of MSG.

THE SAD STATE OF THE STANDARD AMERICAN DIET

While the human brain is largely formed by the age of three, our brains need optimum nutrition throughout our lifetime to maintain brain health, help manufacture healthy brain cells that replace dying ones, and to ward off brain diseases. Let's consider some other ways that Standard American Diet (SAD) is contributing to brain disease.

A Sweet Life?

Sugar is not the harmless substance many people believe it to be, especially in high doses. The average North American consumes 149 pounds of sugar every year. Stack 149 one-pound bags up in your kitchen and you'll have a good idea just how much that is. You will barely have room for anything else.[6]

When hearing this statistic, most people can't believe that they could actually be eating that much sugar. They immediately assume someone else must be making up for them. While that may be possible, it is not very likely. Even if you rarely consume desserts, you may be surprised to learn some of the ways that sugar sneaks itself into your diet. Of course, there are all the obvious places like soft drinks (the average North American drinks 486 twelve-ounce cans of soda pop every year; each one contains about eleven teaspoons of sugar), ice cream, cake, and cookies.[7]

Nancy Appleton, author of *Lick the Sugar Habit,* found sugar hiding in some of the most surprising places: hamburgers, which are injected with sugar to prevent shrinkage; other types of meat, since many meat packers feed sugar to animals prior to slaughter to supposedly improve the flavour and colour of meat; and juice, which may not contain any juice at all. Instead, juice may simply be a storehouse of sugar, colours, and artificial flavours. Most prepared foods contain sugar: canned salmon is typically glazed with sugar prior to canning. Sugar is also used in the processing of luncheon meats, bacon, and canned meats. Sugar is found in bouillon cubes and powders, nuts, peanut butter, and most dry cereals. Even some salt contains sugar! Most condiments contain plentiful amounts of sugar."

Our addiction to sugar is also playing a role in impaired brain function and health.

Refined sugar, in the large doses with which we consume it, may be one of the worst poisons we put into our bodies. Sugar blocks your body's immune response for between four and six hours. That means your body is more likely to fall prey to the thousands of viruses, bacteria, and other infectious diseases present in our environment and in our bodies during that time. While we are quick to blame those pesky pathogens, we rarely look to that decadent triple chocolate cake or that scrumptuous sundae. How could anyone fault something that looks and tastes so sweet?

Research shows that both sugar and alcohol inhibit white blood cell activity. The amount of sugar in one soft drink will lessen white blood cell activity within thirty minutes and normal activity will not resume for four to five hours. The proper functioning of white blood cells is integral to a healthy immune system. You are more vulnerable to bacterial and viral infections after consuming sweets because your white blood cells are unable to function properly to fight these foreign invaders."[8]

Some Symptoms Linked to Sugar Consumption

- Aggression
- Allergies (including those that affect the brain and its normal functioning)
- Anxiety, difficulty concentrating and mood swings in children
- Anxiety in adults
- Atherosclerosis
- Behavioural problems
- Blood platelet adhesiveness, which causes blood clots
- Cardiovascular disease
- Decline in mental capacity
- Depression
- Difficulty concentrating and fatigue
- Emotional problems, depression, mood swings
- Exacerbated symptoms of multiple sclerosis
- Food allergies
- Free radical formation in the bloodstream
- Headaches, including migraines
- Impaired DNA structure
- Increased delta, alpha, and theta brain waves, which can alter the mind's ability to think clearly

- Interference with protein absorption due to changes in the structure of protein
- Ischemic heart disease
- Mental illness
- Raised levels of serotonin, which can narrow blood vessels[9]

This is Your Brain on Artificial Sweeteners

Some people turn to artificial sweeteners hoping to lessen their sugar consumption. Unfortunately, aspartame, and saccharin, and the myriad other artificial sweeteners are even worse. Countless studies show that they are powerful health destroyers. Artificial sweeteners are synthetic chemicals your body has to break down, chemicals your body may find impossible to break down, chemicals that your body was never designed to digest. According to Lynne Melcombe, author of *Health Hazards of White Sugar*, aspartame's effects can be mistaken for Alzheimer's disease, chronic fatigue syndrome, epilepsy, Epstein-Barr virus, Huntington's chorea, hypothyroidism, Lou Gehrig's disease, Lyme disease, Meniere's disease, multiple sclerosis, post-polio syndrome, and sensitivity to mercury amalgam fillings.[10]

Symptoms Linked to Artificial Sweeteners

- Anxiety attacks
- Birth defects, such as mental disabilities
- Brain tumors
- Depression and emotional problems
- Dizziness
- Epilepsy and other seizures
- Fatigue
- Headaches
- Hyperactivity
- Learning disabilities
- Memory loss
- Migraines
- Numbness of extremities

- Psychiatric disorders
- Slurred speech

Hydrogenated and Trans Fats

Trans fats are harmful to every cell in your body, but especially to your brain and the brains of unborn children. Trans fats are incorporated into cellular membranes, including brain and nerve cell membranes, by standing in for healthy fats. The result is impaired brain cells. Brain cell membranes need to be pliable to allow their fluid-like properties to function properly. Research shows that linoleic acid (one type of fat) is over three times wider than the trans-fat form of linoleic acid. As a result, researchers speculate that the blood-brain barrier will leak if it is made up of trans fats, which could allow greater quantities of toxins to access the brain than if it were made of healthy fats. J. Robert Hatherhill found that brain cell membranes made up of trans fats may increase aluminium uptake into the brains of older individuals.[11] His research also indicates that this increased permeability of the blood-brain barrier allows viruses greater access to the brain, may impair the brain-messenger receptors on the surface of brain cells, disrupt signals in the brain, and cause brain cells to become dysfunctional thereby promoting cognitive decline. [12]

What's worse is that people who are deficient in healthy Omega-3 fatty acids will absorb up to twice as many trans fats when they eat them.[13] If you think you're not eating trans fats or hydrogenated fats, here's just a sampling of the places they lurk: margarine, crackers, cookies, pies, vegetable shortening, snack foods, prepared and packaged salad dressings, doughnuts, or french fries. That includes most restaurant foods.

If you're using many grocery store oils, you may unknowingly be subjecting yourself to harmful fats that are already rancid or overheated. Many grocery store oils have been heated to temperatures in excess of five hundred degrees before they even sit on shelves. Every oil has a unique "smoke point," which is the hottest temperature it can be heated to before it becomes denatured and has ill effects on the body. The oil you purchase may have already been overheated prior to its arrival on grocery store shelves. If you're cooking with these oils you may unknowingly be subjecting your brain to harmful fats, from which it will make damaged cellular membranes.

Extra virgin olive oil is one of the rare exceptions to this rule as it is often extracted without high temperatures. But other vegetable oil, canola oil, sunflower oil, safflower oil, and the many other seemingly healthy options may be harming your brain. I'll discuss healthier cooking oil options in an upcoming chapter.

FOOD ADDITIVES

I often ask people, "How many pounds of chemical food additives do you think you eat in a year? The answers vary from one-half pound to five pounds typically. The average person eats 124 pounds of food additives every year.[14] And with names like FD&C Blue No. 1, allyl anthranilate, isopulego, linalyl benzoate, methyl delta-ionone, sodium benzoate, monosodium glutamate, or Yellow dye No. 5, it sounds more like the laboratory analysis at a toxic waste dump than an ingredient list for tonight's dinner.

There are more than three thousand additives and preservatives found in our food supply today.[15] Foods are inundated with artificial colours, flavours, flavour enhancers, bleach, texture agents, conditioners, acid/base balancers, ripening gases, waxes, firming agents, agents that enrich nutrients, preservatives, heavy metals, and other chemicals. Most of these artificial ingredients have never been subjected to long-term tests to determine their effects on human beings. Worse, they are rarely tested to determine the effects on children, whose bodies and brains are developing.

I ask many of my clients to consider a simple question, "Is a small amount of rat poison still rat poison?" The answer of course is a definitive yes. However, many companies in the food industry would answer "no" to that question. How do I know this? Simple. Every day, countless companies manufacture food using small amounts of toxic chemicals. But a small amount of a toxic chemical does not change that it is still toxic, or that synthetic chemicals and altered natural chemicals are not meant to be consumed at all.

Food colours have been shown to cross the blood-brain barrier.[16] The term "barrier" actually instills a false sense of security because chemicals like food dyes actually trick the brain into allowing their entry, putting them in a position to do harm to perhaps the most delicate organ in your body.[17]

EDUCATION OR INDOCTRINATION?

Fast food and processed food dispensers line the halls and cafeterias of schools across Canada and the United States. School administrators willingly accept the combined millions of dollars earned from these artificial foods as part of the schools coffers, justifying the fact that these food items are linked with damage to children's developing brains because the money goes into "activities for the children." Shouldn't children's lifelong health be a higher priority than the amount of cash the school can earn for its programs?

The food processing industry spends millions to target children as part of its overall marketing schemes. After all, they chime in, isn't the school making money for programs for the children? And it's normal to drink a litre or two of cola a day, isn't it? It may be common, but the human body was never designed for soft drinks, trans fats, fried foods, artificial flavours, colours, or any of the other junk that the food industry inundates us with.

No matter what the slick advertisements or product packaging might suggest, there really is no such thing as a free lunch, especially where food additives are concerned. I fear that children and adults alike are ingesting well over one hundred pounds per year of these potentially harmful chemical additives while these substances are still in the experimental stage. I worry that the research documenting their effects on brain health will arrive long after too many children and adults have suffered at the hands of the food processing industry. This large-scale experiment with the very stuff that determines our health or disease state, namely our food supply, needs to end.

THE NOT-SO-RECOMMENDED DAILY ALLOWANCE OF NEUROTOXIC FOOD

Nature, in its infinite wisdom, designed the human body to perform many functions on the food you ingest. At the same time, nature designed the whole foods that will become the cells, tissues, and organs in our bodies. Interfering with natural, whole foods, and the resulting bodily processes that depend on the essential nutrients whole foods are supposed to contain, will have detrimental health effects.

Food is supposed to nourish our brains and bodies, not attack them with harmful chemicals and chemically altered ingredients. The regulatory agencies are starting to demand labelling on trans fats, an inadequate response to the serious harm these fats are causing countless people. But, they've done nothing to stop MSG from being added to foods, even infant foods and so-called health foods. They've done nothing to pull aspartame and other synthetic sweeteners from the shelves. At the same time, the incidence of brain disease soars to incomprehensible heights.

You can take your brain health into your own hands. Now that you are aware of the many sources of neurotoxins, you can begin to eliminate or lessen your exposure to them.

Foods and Supplements High in Neurotoxins

- Antacids, which are frequently taken as digestive and calcium supplements
- Any food containing artificial sweeteners like aspartame
- Any food containing MSG
- Any food made with hydrogenated oils or trans fats
- Calcium supplements containing lead
- Commercially grown foods high in pesticide residues
- Farmed salmon, predatory fish like shark, trout, and swordfish
- Fried and high-fat foods, and many cooking oils found in grocery stores

- Highly processed foods containing food additives or metals
- Shellfish
- Soda pop, which now replaces water for many people and contains excessive sugar
- Vitamin C containing aluminum

The consumption of processed or packaged foods, and foods laden with synthetic food additives and chemically altered ingredients, is clearly a detriment to brain health. While the food manufacturing industry benefits financially from their use, these chemicals are not suitable for human consumption. They are damaging to adult brains and pose an even more alarming threat to the brains of developing fetuses, infants, and children. Our desire for quick and convenient foods shortchanges our brain health. It's time to get back to eating real food. I'll help you do that in the coming chapters.

PART

The Brain Defenders

chapter
5

A Gut Instinct for Brain Health

"Learn to let your intuition—gut instinct—tell you when the food, the relationship, the job isn't good for you, and conversely, when what you're doing is just right."

~ Oprah Winfrey

■ ■ ■ ■ ■ ■ ■

In chapter 5, "A Gut Instinct for Brain Health," you will learn

- that you are what you eat, digest, absorb, and assimilate and what that means to your brain health;
- the fundamentals of digestion;
- how your bowels are essential to the state of health or disease of your brain;
- how bacteria can help you protect your brain;
- which probiotics best support brain health;
- which foods support healthy microflora in your intestines;
- why the state of your liver is so important to your brain health; and
- how to improve your digestion.

■ ■ ■ ■ ■ ■ ■

The last few chapters helped you to make choices to lessen your exposure to substances that may potentially harm the brain; the next few chapters will introduce you to some of the most powerful natural medicines to help you avert brain disease. Somehow, we often equate the term "natural" with "not very effective," but the next few chapters will show you that couldn't be further from the truth. In reality, probiotics (you'll learn what they are momentarily), foods, and herbs are the most potent protectors of your brain's health. And, that's not all. Extensive research continually demonstrates that, like foods and herbs, probiotics also contain substances that can reverse inflammation and damage to the brain.

Your best defence against brain disease lines the produce, spice, and herbal aisles of your grocery or natural food store. Adding these items to your grocery cart could be one of the best decisions you'll ever make to protect your brain against Alzheimer's, Parkinson's, depression, stroke, and other diseases. Yet, what could be simpler? Understanding why foods, spices, herbs, and supplements protect your brain is a tremendous motivator to add these brain-builders to your daily life. Let's get started.

What if I told you that there is another organ system in your body that is intricately linked to the health of your whole body, including your brain? What if I told you that the state of health or disease of this organ system plays a tremendous role in determining your likelihood of suffering from brain disease? What if I told you that this system plays a significant role in your immune system? Now, what if I told you this organ system is your intestines? It may sound hard to believe, but it's true.

There are two main reasons why what happens in your gut plays a significant role in the health of your brain:

1. You are what you eat, according to the old adage. But, "you are what you digest, absorb, and assimilate" is an important addition to the saying. After all, what you eat, digest, absorb, and assimilate will become the building blocks of every cell in your body, including those in your brain. If the digestion process is impaired, your body will lack adequate building blocks to maintain healthy brain and nervous system cells.

2. Research shows that the gastrointestinal (GI) tract plays a huge part in your body's immune response. The GI tract is

one of the main determinants of the levels of inflammation in your body, and whether your body will attack healthy tissue.

Let's take a quick look at the digestion process so you'll better understand how what you eat becomes your cells.

DIGESTION 101

Digestion begins in the mouth. The act of chewing stimulates the secretion of digestive juices, both in the mouth as well as lower in the digestive tract. The saliva in the mouth contains an enzyme called amylase that starts the digestion of starchy foods like pasta, rice, potatoes, or bread. Your mother may have told you to "chew your food well"—she was right. Foods need time to mingle with this enzyme to be properly broken down. If you gulp your food down quickly you are missing a vital stage of the digestion process.

Once you swallow, the food travels down the esophagus to the stomach. The stomach secretes a powerful acid that starts the digestion of protein-based foods like meat, fish, legumes, dairy products, nuts, and seeds. This acid is so powerful that it would burn a hole through your skin if it were located anywhere but the stomach. The stomach contains a thick coat of mucus that acts as a barrier.

After food leaves the stomach, it passes into the small intestines, where other digestive enzymes help break it down further. The pancreas secretes many enzymes into the small intestines to aid in the digestive process. The gall bladder secretes bile—a digestive juice produced by the liver—into the small intestines to assist with fat digestion and to stimulate the intestines to move waste products out of the body.

In the small intestines, nutrients (or toxins, depending on the state of health or disease of your intestines) are absorbed through the intestinal wall into the bloodstream. Without regular bowel movements (after every meal), toxic waste starts to accumulate on the walls of the bowels and is absorbed into the blood. It may even prevent nutrients from being absorbed.

Then, the remaining food is passed down to the large intestine. At this point, the waste matter is mostly liquid. The water passes through the wall of the large intestine to be absorbed by the body. The remaining waste product of the food is then eliminated.

Food molecules that are absorbed through the intestinal walls are transferred to the liver by the bloodstream. There, some food molecules are broken down further while others are converted into fuel that can be stored by the body.

When the intestines are not kept "flushed" of toxic residue and build-up, this fecal matter, along with the accompanying toxins and harmful bacteria, can be re-absorbed into the bloodstream where it can travel throughout the body. This is because vitamins and minerals that are extracted from food are absorbed through the walls of the intestines. If waste matter is backed up in the intestines, waste and the toxins it contains is absorbed instead of nutrients. Not only does your body become self-intoxicating, but also the body cannot adequately take up the nutrients it needs for maintaining health.[1]

Toxic build-up in the intestines can result in virtually any health problem by simply allowing toxins to travel throughout the body via the bloodstream, and by preventing nutrients from being absorbed from food AND SUPPLEMENTS. That's right. If your intestines are backed up, no amount of pill-popping is going to mean good health. You can pop all the calcium or vitamin C, or any other vitamin or mineral supplement you want but your body will not be able to absorb it.[2]

Over one trillion bacteria of more than four hundred different species reside in your intestines.[3] Actually, there are more micro-organisms found in your digestive tract than there are cells in your body.[4] Most of these bacteria reside in the large intestine, which is also known as the colon. We tend to become alarmed at the very thought of bacteria residing in our bodies, but these bacteria are an important part of our health. They help ensure that food is adequately broken down, nutrients are synthesized and absorbed, toxins are not absorbed into the blood, harmful bacteria stay in check, and that the immune system is healthy. These beneficial bacteria are also known as "flora," "micro-flora," and "probiotics" (the opposite of antibiotics).

Naturally-minded health professionals have known for years that plentiful amounts of beneficial flora are imperative to good digestive health, the prevention of autoimmune disorders, and overall health and well-being. But, newer research is connecting intestinal flora to the health of the brain.

THE ENDLESS BENEFITS OF FRIENDLY BACTERIA

The two main types of beneficial bacteria, which are also called "friendly bacteria," include lactobacilli and bifidobacteria. Research is beginning to show that these two types of microflora can lower the levels of toxic compounds that could have detrimental effects on the brain.

Studies show that these bacteria lower negative immune system compounds, called "cytokines," not only in the gut, but also throughout the bloodstream. Cytokines are linked to anxiety, symptoms of depression, and cognitive disturbances when induced in healthy adults.[5] Cytokines also lower levels of an important brain and nerve cell protector.

Lactobacilli and bifidobacteria can also act as antioxidants in the body. Alan C. Logan, ND, FRSH, in his book, *The Brain Diet*, cites four studies that demonstrate probiotics' protective ability against free radical damage, especially against damage to the fatty component of cells. If you recall our discussion about the high level of fat in the brain and the role of free radical damage in various brain diseases, you'll understand why this research is so important to brain health. Free radicals are highly reactive molecules that result from normal metabolic processes, harmful toxins, and other substances. They cause damage to otherwise healthy tissue in the brain and elsewhere in the body, depending on where free radicals are found. Free radicals cause oxidative stress and have been linked to virtually all diseases and the aging process. They speed up aging and disease.

In the *American Journal of Clinical Nutrition*, Swedish researchers showed that oral administration of a strain of lactobacillus plantarum, resulted in a thirty-seven percent reduction in chemicals that mark oxidative stress in the body and are elevated in many brain and neurological diseases. In the same study, the group of people taking a strain of lactobacillus bulgaricus also had a forty-two percent reduction in a particular type of inflammatory cytokines.

Some types of bifidobacteria decline with age. This decline in beneficial bacteria can result in higher levels of harmful bacteria like bacteroides and clostridium. These harmful bacteria are linked with protein by-products that have neurotoxic effects on the brain.

Nonetheless, the University of Tokyo found that the overall levels of bifidobacteria found in the intestines of rural residents of the Yazurihara and Yamanashi regions of Japan were higher than the levels of the same bacteria in urban residents of Tokyo twenty years their junior. Since the oldest living people on the planet are found in Japan, their high vegetable diet warrants serious consideration.

How to Keep the Friendly Flora Thriving

An overgrowth of yeasts, including candida albicans, can result in the production of inflammatory compounds in the intestines, which may in turn be linked to inflammation throughout the body. There are at least 150 species of yeasts known as candida, but the one that frequently tends to become overgrown in the intestines is candida albicans. Overgrowth of this yeast is called "candidiasis." Candida releases over eighty known toxins in the intestines, and causes the membranes of the intestines to become leaky, allowing toxins, bacteria, yeasts, and fecal matter from the intestines to be absorbed into the bloodstream. It is essential to keep these yeasts in balance, and science continues to have breakthroughs that show us how. Imagine that your intestines provide the dance floor for a microscopic dance between the good and bad bugs. If one side takes over the dance floor, there's no room for the others to survive. That's why keeping candida in check is so critical, otherwise they hog the dance floor and prevent the good bacteria from having room to work.

Dr. Logan cites an important Japanese study in his book, *The Brain Diet*. He explains, "Japanese researchers showed that among three different diets (one high in Omega-6 corn oil, another high in beef fat, and a third high in fish oil), it was the fish oil group that showed a beneficial effect on intestinal flora. Specifically, the fish oil diet led to a threefold increase in bifidobacteria and the lowest levels of the bacteroides group of bacteria. This is significant because bacteroides are implicated in cancer."[6] Bifidobacteria are beneficial bacteria while bacteroides have potentially harmful effects in humans.

Test-tube research shows fish oils and flaxseed oils increase beneficial lactobacilli and decrease harmful bacteroides. Olive oil, like its healthy flax and fish oil counterparts, has also been linked with increased beneficial bacteria. It appears that these healthy oils have the potential to increase the beneficial bacteria's ability to adhere to the intestinal walls.

According to research conducted by Dr. Alfred D. Steinberg, at the US National Institute of Health, fish oil is also an effective anti-inflammatory agent. Fish oil acts directly on the immune system by suppressing forty to fifty-five percent cytokine release.

Fish oil, flax oil, and olive oil are not the only foods that increase bifidobacteria growth. Green tea, a common drink in Japan and one that is growing in popularity in North America due to its many healing properties, is also showing promise in its capacity to increase the effectiveness of drugs used to treat candida albicans, while improving populations of healthy bifidobacteria.

Other foods like ginger and honey also appear to benefit the microflora in our intestines. Both foods appear to inhibit harmful bacteria while promoting the growth of beneficial strains like bifidobacteria and lactobacilli. You'll learn more about the other brain-enhancing properties of these foods in the next chapter.

The bacteria helicobacter pylori (or H pylori) which has been linked to stomach ulcers, has also been associated with a greater risk for Alzheimer's disease among other health problems. However, research shows that foods like broccoli sprouts, wasabi (Japanese horseradish), and other vegetables in the brassica family inhibit H pylori while leaving the beneficial bacteria alone. Dr. Logan cites research in the *European Journal of Internal Medicine* that links low-level, chronic inflammation with H pylori. He also cites four research studies that demonstrate various strains of probiotic bacteria can inhibit the growth of H pylori.[7]

In chapter 7, "Healing Herbs," you'll also learn more about herbs that can help kill harmful intestinal yeasts and bacteria.

GREAT DIGESTION MEANS GREAT BRAIN HEALTH

Regardless of the brain disease you may be suffering with, or if you are simply trying to protect your brain from brain disease, it is imperative to improve your digestion and elimination. As we have seen, poor digestion can contribute to an overgrowth of harmful bacteria and yeasts. Optimal digestion can assist healthy microflora in keeping the bowels, immune system, and the brain in better health.

There are many causes of poor digestion in our society, including failure to chew food properly—this is usually caused by eating too quickly. Because the rest of the digestive system depends on food being properly chewed, inadequate chewing may result in indigestion or other uncomfortable symptoms later.

Another cause of poor digestion is drinking large amounts of fluids with meals. Drinking too much at mealtimes dilutes the digestive secretions thereby reducing their efficiency. When food has been adequately broken down by the acid medium in the stomach, the stomach becomes slightly less acidic. This is a signal the body uses to inform the stomach that its job is done. Drinking with meals can improperly "trick" the stomach into "thinking" it has finished digestion because the fluids dilute the acid. This makes the stomach dump the food prematurely into the small intestines. The small intestines cannot perform the work of the stomach. Only the stomach can do the stomach's work.

Eating large and/or complex meals also negatively impacts on digestion. The digestive system was not designed for many of the heavy and complex meals we eat. The larger the meal, the less likely the body can digest it properly. Also, consider what you may have learned in high school chemistry. Because proteins require an acid medium and carbohydrates (starches) require an alkaline medium for digestion, mixing the two can neutralize the digestive juices required for each. The result: inadequate digestion.

Stress also affects digestion. Emotional or mental stress impairs the function of the digestive system. That is why it is best not to eat when you are upset.

Late meals are hard to digest. Because digestive processes lessen in the later part of the day, eating late can ensure that the body does not adequately digest meals. Some of the main problems with eating late include weight gain, gas heartburn, indigestion, and bloating.

Low stomach acid and/or digestive secretions impair digestion. As we age, we tend to produce fewer digestive enzymes and less hydrochloric acid in the stomach. This inadequacy results in improper digestion and digestive problems, along with other health concerns such as allergies, flatulence, weight gain, and nutrient deficiencies.

Another inhibitor of digestion is an overgrowth of harmful bacteria in the intestines. Harmful bacteria overgrowth impedes the healthy flora needed in the intestines to ensure proper nutrient absorption from food.

Conversely, by improving your digestion, you are setting up the fundamentals for better health throughout your body and brain.

■ ■ ■ ■ ■ ■ ■

Tips to Improve Your Digestion

It need not be difficult to improve your digestion. The overall health results of making a few changes to how, when, and what you eat will astound you. Not only will you have less indigestion, flatulence, constipation, diarrhea, or other digestive difficulties, you'll also find other negative symptoms improve, and you'll be creating the necessary conditions for a healthier brain and mental functioning. The reason is simple: you'll absorb more nutrients and fewer waste products into your bloodstream. Fewer waste products in your bloodstream means less inflammation.

1. Chew, chew, chew your food. Then, chew it more.
2. Don't drink with meals. Or, if you have supplements to take with meals, drink a small amount of water.
3. Try simplifying your meals. Stop eating concentrated

protein foods like meat with carbohydrates at the same meal. This is a habit that can take time to change. We've learned that a meal is not complete unless it contains a protein and a starch, such as sandwiches, meat and potatoes, spaghetti and meatballs. However, choosing protein or a starch and completing the meal with a plate of vegetables or a salad is much healthier for your digestion. It gets easier with time and your body will love you for your efforts. Plus, you'll feel more energetic (digestion takes a huge amount of energy) and less bloated. Also, wait a few hours before eating a dessert or fruit (carbohydrates) if you've eaten a protein meal. There isn't a lot of research in the area of simplifying meals, but thousands of people have reported positive results when they make the effort to do this.

4. Try to create a peaceful state of mind when you eat. Stress can disrupt digestion so it is important to try to find some inner calm when eating. If you're constantly in a state of stress, turn to page 185 for some great techniques on stress reduction. If you're prone to eating at your desk, try to leave work behind for a short time while you eat.

5. Eat prior to seven or seven thirty in the evening. That gives your body time to digest foods thoroughly, and to focus on absorption, assimilation, and regeneration, as opposed to digestion, while you sleep.

6. Increase the amount of digestive enzymes in your system. Supplement your diet with a full-spectrum digestive enzyme product. It should contain a wide range of enzymes since each one serves a unique purpose. For example, lipase aids fat digestion, protease aids protein digestion, amylase assists with carbohydrate digestion, lactase assists with digestion of dairy sugars, cellulase and hemicellulase assist with breaking down plant fibre. Ideally, you should get all of these enzymes in a supplement. Always take a digestive enzyme product with each meal. The other way to get more enzymes and to aid digestion is to eat raw foods with every meal. Raw foods

contain enzymes that are destroyed by cooking, canning, processing, and pasteurising food at temperatures over 118 degrees Fahrenheit. Raw foods help lessen the toll on your digestive enzymes. I recommend eating a large salad at least once a day. Snacking on raw fruit is also helpful to increase your intake of enzyme-rich food. Vary the types and ingredients to get a wide range of nutrients and enzymes.

7. Replenish healthy intestinal flora (thereby killing off harmful ones) by supplementing with a probiotic formula. Ideally your probiotic formula should contain a range of intestinal flora including lactobacillus acidophilus, bifidobacterium bifidus, and other lactobacilli such as L bulgaricus and L plantarum. By regulating intestinal flora, you will also regulate bowel movements. This is critical to great health since waste products that pass through the intestines slowly, pass through the walls of the intestine and are absorbed by the blood.

※ ※ ※ ※ ※ ※ ※

LOVE YOUR LIVER

The liver and gall bladder help to determine the state of health or disease of the brain through their ability to neutralize toxins and assist the intestines in eliminating toxins from the body so they do not circulate in the blood, increase the body's inflammatory response, or enter the brain.

The liver is a relatively large organ that sits beneath the ribcage on the right side of the body. With over five hundred functions, it has more jobs than any other organ in the body. It is critical to good health that the liver function up to par. The liver has the task of metabolising fats, carbohydrates, and proteins. It also metabolises hormones, foreign chemicals, and wastes that are created within your body as a by-product of day-to-day living. The liver produces blood-clotting factors and helps with the assimilation and storage of fat-soluble vitamins, which are some of the important antioxidants that protect the brain. In addition to these vitamins, the liver stores carbohydrates and minerals. This powerhouse organ also helps to regulate blood sugar levels by storing excess blood sugar as a substance called "glycogen," which can be released and converted into glucose (sugar) for energy when your body needs it.

The gallbladder is an organ that looks like a small bag tucked beneath the liver. Connected to the liver and an area between the stomach and the intestines, the gall bladder collects bile from the liver and pumps it into the intestines as needed. Bile is a liquid that assists with the removal of waste products from the intestines and helps break down fat.

Detoxification of the liver, in its simplest terms, is divided into two phases, aptly named "Phase 1" and "Phase 2." Either or both phases can be hindered by toxic build-up in the body. Toxins initially enter Phase 1, during which time they are broken down into smaller fragments to allow easier elimination. Then, these fragments pass to Phase 2 in the liver, where enzymes convert toxins to more water-soluble forms or molecules (such as glutathione, glycine, and sulfate). Enzymes are added to toxins to create substances that are less toxic to the body so they can be eliminated in the bile, urine, or stool.

Phase 1 can be hindered if too many toxins enter the liver at once. Phase 2 can often be inefficient at keeping up with the toxins leaving Phase 1, thereby creating an imbalance that often results in symptoms of drug or environmental chemical intolerances. In such cases, people may have trouble with perfumes (after all, they are mostly made up of synthetic and toxic chemicals), gas fumes, paint, or other chemicals.

If the liver is overloaded with toxins, these toxins can leave the liver to be stored in fat tissue, central nervous system cells, and even the brain. These stored toxins may circulate in the blood at other times, contributing to chronic disease.[8]

It is important to eat foods that help the liver to detoxify, thereby neutralizing and eliminating many toxins that could otherwise have damaging effects on the brain. Supportive herbs known for their liver-boosting properties are also beneficial to improve the liver's capacity to deal with the growing number of toxins it is subjected to. You'll find a list of liver supportive foods in chapter 6 and specific herbs to improve the liver's toxin elimination capacity in chapter 7.

You are what you eat, digest, absorb, and assimilate. By improving your digestion and elimination, you'll be making big strides in improving your overall health and especially your brain health. While we tend to fragment our bodies into parts when we think of our health, a more holistic view considers how everything functions together for optimum health. When you take into consideration what's happening with your digestion and the state of your bowels, you are paying attention to a critical link in your journey toward optimum brain health.

chapter
6

Protective Foods and Nutrients

"One cannot think well, love well, or sleep well if one has not dined well."

~ Virginia Wolf

■ ■ ■ ■ ■ ■ ■

In chapter 6, "Protective Foods and Nutrients," you will learn

- how the food you eat affects your brain health;
- why it is important to give your brain an "oil change";
- the pros and cons of protein;
- the best brain-building carbohydrates;
- how to cook gluten-free grains;
- the best brain-building nutrients and how they affect brain health;
- my Top Twenty Brain Superfoods; and
- My Top Five Supplement Picks for Just About Everyone.

■ ■ ■ ■ ■ ■ ■

Don't be fooled by nature's beautiful packaging and delicious taste, food can be more powerful than pharmaceutical drugs in protecting the brain against disease. Your body's greatest weapons in the war against brain disease come in the form of power foods like berries, nuts, grapes, green tea, garlic, and many other common foods and spices. Specific nutritional supplements are also potent brain boosters that should be considered as part of any brain disease prevention program. This chapter will explain the many foods and nutrients you should consider. There is no need to try to memorize everything listed below, since chapter 8 will organize all this information into a simple plan. With some of the nutrients suggested, I will offer recommended amounts to take, while in other cases (like with foods), there's no need to worry about amounts.

While it is important to enjoy the taste of foods, it is even more important to eat foods that provide nutritional value and help prevent disease. The great news is that you don't have to choose between the two. Many people find it hard to believe that healthy, nutritious food can taste great. But it can.

The foods you eat affect brain function in numerous ways: foods assist with the manufacturing of brain hormones called neurotransmitters that enhance memory, concentration, and reaction time; foods provide energy for the development and repair of healthy brain cells.

Some foods even contain potent substances that actually cross the blood-brain barrier to protect the brain from environmental toxins, others lessen free radicals in the body before they can make their way to the brain, and still others lessen inflammation in the brain and body. Almost daily, new studies are released that indicate the miraculous properties of fruits, veggies, spices, and herbs that prevent or treat brain disease.

Let's explore the many delicious brain-boosting foods and the important nutrients required to provide the brain with energy and nutrition to make healthy brain cells and brain hormones, while they protect your brain against harmful pollutants, free radicals, and inflammation.

The main classifications for the various nutrients required by your brain are macronutrients and micronutrients.

MACRONUTRIENTS

Types of Macronutrients

- Amino acids from protein foods
- Essential fatty acids from fats
- Fibre
- Sugars from carbohydrates (carbs)

Give Your Brain an Oil Change

About sixty percent of your brain is fat and, as I mentioned earlier, your body is constantly creating new cells to replace old, worn-out ones. That means that you need to get adequate fat from your diet. But, not just any fat will do. Some fats damage the brain. The Standard American Diet (SAD) worsens inflammation in the body, and this inflammation can damage delicate brain tissues. These unhealthy fats are trans fats, hydrogenated fats, and most saturated fats found in fried foods, shortening, lard, margarine, and foods made with these items.

The typical diet, if it contains any essential fatty acids, usually includes fats found in meat and poultry, or healthier fats from nuts and seeds called Omega-6 fatty acids.

Other fats help keep the lining of brain cells flexible so that memory and other brain messages can pass easily between cells.[1] Both Omega-6 and Omega-3 fats are important to brain health and should be eaten in a one-to-one or two-to-one ratio to each other. However, the average North American eats these foods in a twenty-to-one to a fifty-to-one ratio, causing a huge imbalance and resulting Omega-3 deficiency. In this ratio, Omega-6 fats can cause or worsen inflammation, for which there is insufficient Omega-3 fats to keep inflammation under control.

According to research conducted by Dr. Joseph Mercola, people consumed less than one pound of liquid vegetable oil per year at the turn of the nineteenth century. At the turn of the twentieth century the average person consumed seventy-five pounds of oil per year. Almost all of these oils were loaded in Omega-6 fatty acids, trans fats, or oils that have been turned into solids like hydrogenated fats. So it's not hard to understand why the ratio is so out of proportion now. The oils highest in Omega-6s, the ones you're most likely getting too much of, are corn, soy, canola, safflower, and sunflower.

But, you are more than what *you* eat. I read somewhere that "you are what you eat eats." So that means if you eat a diet with meat or poultry that was fed corn, or other grains high in Omega-6s, you're getting lots of Omega-6s indirectly.

The best sources of Omega-3 fatty acids include flax seeds or oil, olives and olive oil, walnuts and walnut oil, and fatty coldwater fish, particularly wild salmon. Fish and fish oil is one of nature's weapons against Alzheimer's disease. Research shows that the Omega-3 fatty acids found in fish may fend off Alzheimer's. In one study, researchers genetically engineered mice to develop the disease. Mice were divided into two groups: one group was fed a diet rich in docosahexanoic acid (DHA), the type of Omega-3 fatty acid found in coldwater fish. The other group was fed a diet low in these fats. In only five months, researchers found seventy percent less amyloid protein—the plaque that has been implicated in Alzheimer's disease—in mice fed the high DHA diet.[2]

DHA makes up a large part of the lining of brain cells, so it is imperative to eat a diet rich in these Omega-3 fats to keep the cellular lining flexible enough to allow memory messages to pass between cells. DHA promotes nerve transmission in the central nervous system, and protects the energy centres of the cells, called "mitochondria," from damage.

A study of 815 people aged sixty-four to ninety-four published in the *Archives of Neurology* found that people who ate fish one to three times per month had a forty percent lower risk of suffering from Alzheimer's disease than those who never ate fish. Those who consumed fish once a week had a sixty percent lower risk.[3]

Another study in the journal, *Lipids*, showed that people with low levels of Omega-3 fatty acids may have a higher risk of dementia or cognitive impairment, including problems with memory.[4] The same researchers also found low levels of DHA in patients suffering from age-related cognitive decline and Alzheimer's.[5]

This type of research helps us to understand the importance of getting adequate healthy fats in our diet to prevent brain diseases. But, that's not all. Another study in the *Journal of Molecular Neuroscience* showed that increasing DHA fat intake can actually REVERSE some of the mental decline associated with Alzheimer's.[6] That's astounding research that doctors need to start passing along to their patients. As the impressive research on fish oils continues to pile up, DHA supplementation will continue to be one of the natural superstars against brain diseases.

Fish that contain high amounts of this Omega-3 fatty acid include mackerel, sardines, albacore tuna, salmon, lake trout, and herring. But be aware, some of these fish have become contaminated with mercury and, as you just learned in chapter two, some research links mercury to the development of Alzheimer's disease. So, it is important to avoid fish that consistently shows up high on the mercury radar, including predatory fish like swordfish and shark, as well as sea bass, northern pike, tuna, walleye, and largemouth bass. Salmon raised in fish farms also frequently shows up with high amounts of mercury, not to mention that farmed salmon often contains antibiotic residues and lower levels of the important Omega-3 fatty acids.

It is highly advisable for people looking to prevent brain disease, and for those suffering from a brain disorder, to supplement with a high quality, uncontaminated source of fish oil daily. See the resources section of this book for more information about fish oil supplements. Choose one that contains both DHA and EPA, since both are critical to brain health. The good news for people who are deficient of Omega-3 fatty acids: your body will absorb twice as many of these important fats when you start consuming or supplementing with them than people who have adequate amounts. That's your body's wisdom trying to correct a serious imbalance and create better health.

Olives and Olive Oil

The names Moroccan, kalamata, nicoise, picholine, and manzanilla sound almost as good as these varieties of olives taste. Sulphite-free olives are an excellent source of healthy monounsaturated fats and vitamin E. Monounsaturated fats have a beneficial role to play in maintaining the outer membranes of cells and protecting our bodies' genetic material and energy-producing cellular components, mitochondria.

Vitamin E offers antioxidant protection to the fatty components of the brain and can lower the risk of damage and inflammation. This vitamin is also the body's primary fat-soluble antioxidant, meaning that it neutralizes damaging free radicals in all the fat-rich areas of the body, including the brain and the protective coating for the nerves. Like monounsaturated fats, vitamin E also helps protect the energy production centres in the cells to ensure our cells are capable of creating adequate energy for our many bodily processes and brain functions.

Olives and olive oil also help prevent the oxidation of cholesterol. Oxidized cholesterol is linked to stroke.[7] The anti-inflammatory actions of monounsaturated fats, vitamin E, and beneficial plant chemicals called "polyphenols," also found in olives and olive oil, help lessen the likelihood of inflammation in the brain. Olive oil is also rich in Omega-9 fatty acids that are important to the brain.

Because olive oil is extracted from olives, it has the same beneficial properties as olives. However, be sure to use only organic, cold-pressed extra virgin olive oil, since it retains more of the beneficial nutrients and lacks potentially harmful pesticides. When cooking with any type of oil, including olive oil, it is important to be sure that the oil never smokes. If it does, it has reached the "smoke point" which is different for every type of oil. The smoke point is the point at which the oil will have a damaging effect on your body. Most types of vegetable oils available in grocery stores have already been heated to over five hundred degrees Fahrenheit during processing, which is well beyond the smoke point, even before it gets to your kitchen. These oils should be completely avoided. Extra virgin olive oil is the rare exception that tends to be processed at lower temperatures and is therefore fine for cooking at low temperatures.

But, it's important to remember when you're cooking with any type of oil: if it smokes while you are heating it, it is essential to throw it out and start over. Otherwise, the heat destroys the benefits of the oil and it becomes capable of damaging cells in your brain through free radicals and inflammatory processes.

Be sure to choose olives that are free from sulphites, as many commercial brands of olives contain sulphites and chemical preservatives.

THE PROS AND CONS OF PROTEIN

Amino acids are the building blocks of protein. While amino acids are required by your brain for optimal health, you need to be sure that your body is able to break down the protein foods you choose. Also, you need to ensure that you're getting the correct amino acids in the right balance. The main amino acids required in adequate amounts by the brain are taurine and glycine. Some of the best sources of taurine include wild game, oatmeal, organic cocoa, eggs, turkey, duck, and avocado. Provided other rich sources of amino acids are included in your diet, your body is able to manufacture adequate amounts of glycine.

Some lesser-known foods that are high in usable protein include avocado, legumes like lentils or kidney beans, nuts, nut butters, almond milk, soy milk, tofu, bean sprouts, and alfalfa sprouts. Most people are shocked to learn that one avocado contains more usable protein than an eight-ounce steak. Also, bean sprouts are loaded with highly absorbable protein, thanks to the enzymes that allow for quick and easy digestion, provided they are eaten raw.

While the brain needs amino acids, too much protein from animal sources, particularly red meat, which is high in saturated fats, can cause inflammation in the body and the brain—a serious threat to brain health.

Getting adequate protein is less of a problem than most people realise. Most foods contain protein and many vegetarian sources of protein are actually superior to animal sources because they are more digestible. However, getting adequate amounts of the *right kinds* of protein does present a problem for many people. The easiest rule of thumb with protein is to limit the amount of acid-inducing animal proteins and include more vegetarian protein sources. That doesn't mean you need to eliminate meat from your diet. Some of the best options include organic turkey, organic chicken, wild game, fish (excluding those high in mercury that we discussed earlier), avocado, quinoa (a grain, pronounced "keen-wah"), raw nuts, sesame seeds, tahini, nut butters, tofu, soy milk, almond milk, and legumes.

Brain-Building Carbs

Healthy carbs provide the sugars that your brain needs for energy. I can almost hear some readers justifying their sugar addictions with that statement. However, your body has specific sugar needs. Refined or concentrated sugars like those found in cola, ice cream, cakes, cookies, or other sugary foods provide a quick sugar rush that just as quickly causes blood sugar levels to plummet. That kind of sugar rollercoaster is detrimental to brain health, not to mention the immune system.

Instead, the brain requires sustained energy from healthy carbs like fruit and whole-grains, and legumes. Yes, legumes are high in protein and carbs, making them an excellent food choice.

Many grains contain a sticky substance called gluten that causes an immune response in sensitive individuals who have inherent gluten sensitivities. Like other sensitivities, gluten sensitivity rarely causes the same symptoms as pollen and environmental allergies. Instead gluten may cause a build-up of inflammation in the body. Since inflammation is linked to many brain diseases and has been identified by many natural health professionals as a causative factor for autism, it is best to avoid or limit your intake of gluten-containing grains. The main ones are wheat (which includes whole wheat or white flour and anything made with them), rye, oats, kamut, and spelt.

Stay clear of "enriched" grain foods as well. Author of *Low Carb Recipes*, Dana Carpender, once told me that "enriched flour products are typically grain products that have had all the fibre and some thirty-five or more nutrients removed and five added back in. Enriched-flour products are comparable to being robbed of all your clothes, money, shoes, and personal belongings while walking to the bus stop. Then, the thief gives you your shoes and a quarter for the bus and tells you that you've been 'enriched' by the experience."

Better sources of gluten-free carbs include brown rice, wild rice, almond flour, tapioca flour, potato flour, arrowroot, or quinoa. Brown rice is more nutritious and a better option than white rice. It offers vitamin E and is high in fibre. Quinoa, a staple of the ancient Incas who revered it as sacred, is not a true grain, rather an herb. It is a complete protein and is high in iron, B-vitamins, and fibre.

Also not a true grain, wild rice is actually a type of aquatic grass seed native to the United States and Canada. It tends to be a bit pricier than other grains, but its high content of protein, and nutty flavour make wild rice worth every penny. It is an excellent choice for people with celiac disease or who have gluten or wheat sensitivities. Add wild rice to soups, stews, salads, and pilaf. It is important to note that wild rice is black. There are many blends of white and wild rice, which tend to consist primarily of refined white rice. Be sure to use only wild rice, not the blends, to avoid refined rice.

Cooking Guide for Gluten-Free Whole Grains

Grain	Amount of Grain	Amount of Water	Cooking Time in Minutes	Yield (Approx)
Quinoa	1 cup	2 cups	15	2 ¾ cups
Rice, Brown	1 cup	2 cups	35–40	2 ¾ cups
Rice, Wild	1 cup	3 cups	50–60	3–4 cups

THE MAIN TYPES OF MICRONUTRIENTS

- Vitamins
- Minerals
- Enzymes
- Phytochemicals

The ABCs of Vitamins

Every cell in your body needs particular vitamins to work properly. Without adequate vitamins, cellular functions begin to break down until there are potentially serious flaws in their workings. If this happens the cells may even die off prematurely as the body tries to protect itself against possible damage. The main vitamins required by brain cells are B-vitamins, especially B6, B12, niacin (B3), and folate (also called B9), vitamin C, and vitamin E.

To B or Not to B (Supplement, That Is)

All B-vitamins are important for the formation of neurotransmitters, the hormones that act as messengers in the brain. These hormones help regulate the many functions of the brain and body, including healthy mood regulation. Most people have some deficiencies of the B-vitamins complex, especially B12, which tends to be more difficult to absorb with age. Since B-complex vitamins work best when combined, they are often sold in combination form in tablets or capsules. Depending on the nature of the brain disorder, specific individual B-vitamins may need to be further supplemented. In that case, it is still best to take a B-complex vitamin and add extra B12 or folic acid, for example. Most people will benefit from supplementation of fifty milligrams of most B-complex vitamins, with the exception of folate and B12, which are measured in micrograms, not milligrams.

As with any nutritional supplement, it is best to work directly with a holistic nutritionist, doctor of natural medicine, or naturopath who can guide you in individualizing your supplement choices to suit your particular needs. He or she can also guide you as to whether you might want to take higher doses of a particular B-complex vitamins.

Niacin

Niacin protects against Alzheimer's disease. It appears to protect the brain by stimulating the production of acetylcholine, which can be destroyed by organophosphates. Niacin is critical for proper activity of the brain chemical acetylcholine.[8] Fifty milligrams is a good dose for someone who is healthy. Higher doses may be required for people suffering from brain diseases. A holistic health professional can assist you with determining higher dosages, if necessary.

B12

All B-vitamins help brain cells communicate with each other by assisting with the production of brain hormones called neurotransmitters, such as serotonin and dopamine. B12 is especially important to help the body produce the neurotransmitter acetylcholine that allows nerve cells to transmit memory signals.

Studies even link a B12 deficiency to an increased risk of Alzheimer's disease or Alzheimer's-like symptoms of memory loss.[9] A study in the journal *Clinical Therapeutics* showed that memory-related symptoms diminished when people received injections of vitamin B12.[10] B12 deficiencies have also been linked to depression, with supplementation being beneficial.[11] Take a B-complex vitamins supplement along with extra B12. A therapeutic dose of B12 for the prevention or treatment of brain disorders including depression is one thousand micrograms.

While the best way to obtain and the most useable form of B-vitamins is from foods that are rich in B-vitamins (eggs, fish, lean meat, legumes, whole grains, and nuts), it is wise to take a B-vitamins complex supplement as well. Alternatively, be sure that your high quality multivitamin contains adequate B-vitamins.

Some people have low levels of a substance called "intrinsic factor" in their stomachs. Intrinsic factor helps with the absorption of B12. If you don't produce adequate intrinsic factor—and the only way to find out is through medical tests—you may benefit from vitamin B12 injections. If you have memory problems and are supplementing with B12 nutritional supplements, you may want to get your doctor to test for an intrinsic-factor deficiency.

Folate

Folate helps protect nerve cells from damage. A study in the journal *Neurology* linked low folate levels to an increased risk of developing Alzheimer's disease.[12] Low levels of folate have also been linked to depression. Four hundred micrograms is often sufficient for preventative purposes, however, for those suffering from depression, Alzheimer's or another brain disorder, eight hundred micrograms is beneficial.

Research was presented at the 2005 Alzheimer's Association meeting in Washington, DC, showing that a high dose (eight hundred micrograms daily) of folic acid daily may slow cognitive decline related to aging. Researchers tested over eight hundred people with good cognitive functioning for three years. Those who were given the supplement scored 5.5 years younger than their age. On tests for cognitive speed, people given the supplement scored as well as people 1.9 years younger. The daily dosage typically recommended is four hundred micrograms.

In numerous studies, B-vitamins, particularly B6, B12, niacin, and folate, demonstrated the ability to lower levels of an artery-hardening chemical called "homocysteine," found in the blood. Excess homocysteine can lead to memory disorders and Alzheimers', according to a study in the *Journal of Nutrition, Health & Aging*.[13]

Vitamins C and E

Two powerful antioxidants used by the brain are vitamins C and E. The *New England Journal of Medicine* reported that vitamin E is more effective in treating Alzheimer's disease than any pharmaceutical drug on the market.[14] Antioxidants like vitamin E are also showing promise in their ability to protect the brain from damage. Additional research found that diets rich in foods containing vitamin E were associated with reduced risk of Alzheimer's disease.[15]

Vitamin E is the best-known antioxidant for its supportive role in maintaining brain and memory function. The *Archives of Neurology* reported that in a group of 2889 adults over the age of sixty-five, those who had the highest vitamin E intake had the lowest rate of cognitive decline. Another study in the *New England Journal of Medicine* showed that people with somewhat severe Alzheimer's disease who supplemented with two thousand IU per day of vitamin E slowed the disease's progression.[16] Other studies found that people with Alzheimer's or dementia have low levels of vitamins C and E.

Foods that are high in vitamin E include whole-grains, almonds, sunflower seeds, and avocados. Foods high in vitamin C include broccoli, red peppers, kiwi, and strawberries.

It is imperative to eat foods rich in antioxidants since they are more beneficial for the body than supplements, but supplementing with additional vitamins C and E is helpful to protect the brain against damaging free radicals.

Current recommendations for fruit and vegetable intake are frighteningly low and do not consider the high nutritional needs of the brain. I highly advise trying to eat at least nine servings of fruits and vegetables daily. A serving is approximately a one-half cup portion. That sounds like a lot, but a piece of fruit or two alongside breakfast, a large green salad for lunch or to accompany lunch, veggies with dinner, and a couple pieces of fruit or vegetable sticks for snacks, and you'll easily find yourself surpassing that amount.

MINERALS: BRAIN-BOOSTERS FROM LAND AND SEA

A deficiency in any mineral may mean less than optimal brain functioning but there are some critical minerals that are especially important for proper brain health, including magnesium, iron, zinc, and selenium.

Magnesium

While there are many minerals that are important to healthy brain functioning, the most important ones are magnesium, iron, and zinc. Based on his research at the Mineral Element, Nutrition, Neuropsychological Function, and Behaviour Research Lab at the Grand Forks Human Nutrition Research Center in North Dakota, James Penland, PhD identifies magnesium as a critical mineral to maintain normal brain activity.[17]

A study published in *Procedures of the North Dakota Academy of Sciences* linked low magnesium intake to poor scores on memory tests in rats. Other research links low magnesium levels to decreased cognitive functioning in humans.

Magnesium is involved with countless biological and chemical functions in the body, particularly in stabilizing brain wave patterns and in increasing blood flow to the brain. Magnesium-rich foods include nuts, legumes, whole grains, avocados, and artichokes.

Pumping Iron and Zinc

Researchers know that iron and zinc play significant roles in the a bility to concentrate; yet, they don't know exactly how these two minerals affect mental functioning. Studies indicate that a slight deficiency will show up as memory and attention span problems, even before a blood test can detect low levels. Zinc is involved in over two hundred functions in the body and is present in almost every cell, including brain cells.

A study published in *Pediatrics* stated that adolescents who were iron-deficient did worse on math tests than did their counterparts with normal levels. Another study found in the *British Journal of Nutrition* found that a zinc deficiency can interfere with communication between brain cells. Additional research by Mary Kretsch, PhD, research physiologist with the government's Western Human Nutrition Research Center in Davis, California, indicates a direct relationship between iron and zinc levels and poor attention and memory. People with the lowest iron and zinc levels also have the greatest cognitive difficulties.[18]

Menstruating women need eighteen milligrams of iron daily, while post-menopausal women require only eight milligrams maximum per day. Women need about eight milligrams of zinc daily as well. Men should strive for eight milligrams of iron and eleven milligrams of zinc daily. Because these minerals are often found in the same foods, they are easiest to obtain together from sources like legumes (including tofu, tempeh, and other soy products), red meat, poultry, and whole-grains.

Selenium

While the mineral selenium is only required in small amounts, it is a powerful antioxidant that helps lessen free radical activity in the body. It helps form an important detoxification enzyme called glutathione peroxidase that works closely with other antioxidant nutrients like vitamins C and E to neutralize free radicals. Many people are deficient in this important mineral due to agricultural techniques that deplete the soil of selenium. Raw walnuts and Brazil nuts are excellent sources of this vital nutrient. Supplementation of one hundred to three hundred micrograms may also be helpful to eliminate brain-destructive free radicals from the body.[19] Keep in mind that selenium in high doses is toxic. Avoid consuming more than nine hundred micrograms per day over a prolonged period of time. Based on research by the National Academy of Sciences, the upper intake of four hundred micrograms may be a better maximum dose.

Iodine

A low thyroid function may underlie many brain disorders, so it is imperative to get adequate amounts of natural iodine in your food to help keep your thyroid balanced. The thyroid gland is in the throat region and produces important hormones that help you feel energetic, balance body temperature, and perform many other important functions. The best sources of thyroid-balancing iodine are sea vegetables, including kelp, hijiki, agar, and nori. Try to eat some sea vegetables daily to benefit from their many minerals, including iodine content.

FIBRE

In addition to assisting with normal bowel functioning, fibre is critical to the health of your brain in other ways.

1. Fibre helps prevent backup in the intestines of waste materials, which otherwise could intoxicate the body by penetrating the intestinal walls into the blood and ultimately end up in the brain. In this way, fibre helps to eliminate waste materials. Those include excess bacterial or yeast overgrowth that can be found in the intestines. Fibre helps to push harmful pathogens out of the body.
2. Fibre also binds to specific toxins in the body to escort them out. Different types of fibre bind to different toxins. For example, wheat bran has been shown to bind with the metals cadmium and mercury; rice bran and spinach fibre binds to PCBs; pectin, carrot, and cabbage fibre binds to the heavy metal lead.[20]

3. Fibre also helps to regulate the release of glucose by preventing rapid blood sugar spikes. This helps to ensure that the brain has a steady supply of energy rather than the energy surges and crashes common to people consuming the Standard American Diet.

Legumes are some of the highest sources of fibre. It is easy to add chickpeas, lentils, kidney beans, navy beans, or other beans to your diet to reap the nutritional benefits they offer. Whole grains like those mentioned above are also excellent sources of fibre. Most fruits and vegetables contain beneficial amounts of fibre, adding one more reason to consume them.

NATURE'S PHYTO PHARMACY AGAINST FREE RADICALS

When it comes to protecting the brain, food is truly the best medicine, if you know which foods to select. With thousands of healing substances found in fruits and vegetables, and more discovered almost daily, adding brain "Superfoods" to your diet is one of the best decisions you can make for your health.

Mother Nature offers protection against free radicals in the form of antioxidants. Antioxidants are powerful nutrients that prevent free radical damage. They are found in many foods, especially green leafy vegetables. The more deeply or brightly coloured the vegetable, typically the greater the number of antioxidants it contains.

The US Department of Agriculture (USDA) developed a scale called the Oxygen Radical Absorbance Capacity, or ORAC, to identify foods that have high levels of antioxidants. Two studies published in the *Journal of Nutrition* and the *American Journal of Nutrition* found that when humans eat high-ORAC fruits and vegetables, the antioxidant power of their blood raises between thirteen and twenty-five percent. Eating high-ORAC foods may help slow the processes associated with aging the brain and body.

Top Antioxidant Foods (ORAC units per one hundred grams)

Prunes	5770
Raisins	2830
Blueberries	2400
Kale	1770
Strawberries	1540
Spinach	1260
Raspberries	1220
Brussels Sprouts	980
Plums	949
Alfalfa Sprouts	930
Broccoli Florets	890
Beets	840
Oranges	750
Red Grapes	739
Red Bell Peppers	710
Cherries	670
Onions	450
Corn	400
Eggplant	390

Additional foods that are nutrient-rich and great for their anti-aging properties include avocados, carrots, cabbage, citrus fruit, green tea, legumes, garlic, seaweed, and tomatoes. All of these foods contain many powerful and potent phytochemicals and antioxidants.

Flavonoids Provide More Than Just Flavour

There are over four thousand substances in plant foods called "flavonoids," also sometimes called "vitamin P," that occur naturally and have tremendous medicinal properties. Colourful fruits and vegetables, like blueberries, strawberries, and spinach, contain a category of flavonoids, called "polyphenols." Polyphenols prevent oxidative damage in the brain. A study of rats fed extracts of blueberries, strawberries, and spinach for eight weeks showed that these potent antioxidant foods reversed some effects of age-related brain decline.[21] Other research shows that flavonoids also work with vitamin C to prevent the vitamin's breakdown in the body, allowing it to continue working as an antioxidant to protect the brain against free radicals.

Spinach—More Than Just for Popeye

In addition to the study above, which showed the brain benefits of spinach, other studies, documented in the *Journal of Neuroscience,* of middle-aged rats fed diets with added spinach, strawberry extract, or vitamin E for nine months found that spinach proved most potent in protecting nerve cells against the effects of aging in two parts of the brain.

Benefits of Blue for Grey Matter

Blueberries contain a group of flavonoids called proanthocyanidins. Proanthocyanidins have a unique capacity to protect both the watery and fatty parts of the brain against damage from some environmental toxins. Proanthocyanidins decrease free radical activity within and between brain cells.[22] Blueberry proanthocyanidins have greater antioxidant properties than vitamins C and E. Blueberries appear to have some of the highest concentrations of these powerful antioxidants.

Other studies show that animals given blueberry extract had less motor skill decline and performed better on memory tests than those not given the extract. Researchers indicated that blueberry extract may reverse some age-related memory loss and motor skill decline.[23]

Blueberries are excellent anti-inflammatory agents. They increase the amounts of compounds called heat-shock proteins that decrease as people age, thereby causing inflammation and damage, particularly in the brain. By eating blueberries regularly, research shows that these heat-shock proteins stop declining and inflammation lessens, not to mention that they just taste fabulous.

Blueberries are turning out to be one of the best brain Superfoods and they are easy to add to your diet. Obviously fresh organic blueberries are best, but frozen blueberries are also great. Frozen blueberries are also tasty as is (after thawing slightly), since they taste like sorbet. Or you can blend frozen blueberries into a smoothie or thaw them and eat whole.

From the Vine to Your Palate

Dr. Egemen Savaskan and colleagues at the University of Basel in Switzerland found a molecule in grapes, grape juice, and red wine which may protect the brain against Alzheimer's disease. Called resveratrol, it is an antioxidant thought to be responsible for many of the purported benefits of red wine on brain cells. The researchers found that resveratrol protected the cells from beta-amyloid-induced oxidative damage by mopping up free radicals. However, resveratrol did not protect the cells from oxidative stress that was not caused by beta-amyloid. Savaskan stresses that though his findings suggest that resveratrol may help to protect against Alzheimer's, it is not a good idea for seniors to drink red wine to ward off the disease since alcohol can be toxic to cells.[24]

Red or purple grapes are a superior source of resveratrol and other flavonoids found in grapes. While you may enjoy eating the seedless kind, even the grape seeds contain valuable phytochemicals with antioxidant powers. You can obtain some of the benefits of the seeds by blending whole grapes with a small amount of water in a high powered blender like a Vita-Mix. This blender grinds the seeds and grapes into a healthy whole grape juice, which is complete with all the nutrients and enzymes of grapes and without the high intake of refined or concentrated sugars found in pre-packaged grape juice.

The Memory-Boosting Power of Tomatoes

Tomatoes contain a powerful memory-boosting phytonutrient called "lycopene." Researchers at the University of Kentucky studied a group of Catholic nuns. Those who consumed at least thirty milligrams of lycopene in their daily diets were 3.6 times more able to take care of themselves physically and had sharper memories than those who didn't consume high amounts of lycopene.[25]

Tea for Two Hemispheres

Researchers found that people who drank two or more cups of tea each day were less likely to develop Parkinson's disease.[26] Another study suggests that regular caffeine exposure may counteract the age-related degenerative process in the brain that leads to loss of the brain chemical dopamine, a key factor in Parkinson's.[27]

Another important group of natural chemicals found in tea are called catechins. These natural phytochemicals are also showing promise as brain protectors.[28]

Green tea contains potent antioxidants with twenty times the power to protect against free radicals than vitamin E. Green tea also lowers the risk of blood clots and clumping linked to stroke. In another study, green tea extract was shown to protect animals from the effects of a neurotoxic agent. Green tea extract reduced neuron loss in the area of the brain that is damaged in Parkinson's disease.[29]

Chicken Soup for the Soul and Chocolate for the Brain

Savour chocolate. The cocoa in it has the same disease-fighting anti-oxidants found in vegetables, according to Eric Gershwin, MD, a professor of medicine at the University of California in Davis.[30] Choose only organic, dark chocolate. Most of the world's supply of chocolate originates in West Africa where harsh pesticides and leaded gasoline are still in use and can contaminate the cacao plants and find its way into your body through the chocolate you consume. Organic dark chocolate is rich in the antioxidants called flavonoids. It's best to avoid bars that tend to be high in sugar since sugar is linked to inflammation in the body. Avoid processed chocolate since it often contains heavy metals, a serious threat to brain health. Instead, purchase pure, unsweetened, organic cocoa and add it to shakes, smoothies, and baking. Yes, it is possible to love the food you eat while still ensuring your brain receives all the nutrients it needs for optimal functioning. Moderation is the key when it comes to chocolate.

Ginger to Counter Inflammation

A study conducted by Dr. Honlei Chen and his colleagues at the Harvard

School of Public Health suggest that inflammation plays an important role, among other things, in the development of Parkinson's disease.[31] Inflammatory processes also appear in the development of Alzheimer's disease. Therefore, foods that have an anti-inflammatory property play an important role in the prevention of brain disease and maintenance of a healthy brain.

Fresh ginger is one of the best natural anti-inflammatory foods. According to Dr. Krishna C. Srivastava of Odense University in Denmark, ginger is superior to non-steroidal anti-inflammatory drugs (NSAIDs) in alleviating inflammation. NSAIDs work on one level, blocking the substances that cause inflammation, while ginger works on at least two mechanisms: ginger blocks the formation of inflammatory compounds; and ginger has antioxidant properties that actually break down inflammation and acidity in the body.[32] This is promising research since anti-inflammatory drugs are being considered for use with inflammation-related brain diseases.

The Anti-Inflammatory Power of Cherries

Muraleedharan Nair, PhD, professor of natural products and chemistry at Michigan State University, found that tart cherry extract is ten times more effective than aspirin at relieving inflammation. Only two tablespoons of the concentrated juice need to be taken daily for effective results. Later she found that sweet cherries, blackberries, raspberries, and strawberries have similar effects.[33]

Munch on Celery to Beat Brain Inflammation

James Duke, PhD, author of *The Green Pharmacy*, found more than twenty anti-inflammatory compounds in celery and celery seeds, including a substance called "apigenin," which is powerful in its anti-inflammatory action. If you're not sure how to use celery seeds, add them to soups, stews, or as a salt substitute in many recipes. One of my favorite appetizers is celery bread instead of garlic bread. Simply brush olive oil on whole grain bread (preferably not wheat) and sprinkle with celery seeds, bake in a 350-degree oven until golden-brown and serve as a tasty side dish.

Tears Get in Your Eyes

US general, Ulysses S. Grant, once stated, "I will not move my army without onions." Perhaps he understood the food's potent medicine. Regular consumption of onions (two or more times per week) has been associated with lower cholesterol and blood pressure levels, both of which help reduce the risk of stroke, among other diseases.[34] The beneficial effects may be associated with the sulphur compounds found in onions, as well as the mineral chromium and vitamin B6, all of which help reduce high levels of homocysteine, a risk factor for stroke. The sulphur compounds are also essential to help your body's main detox organ, the liver, eliminate environmental toxins.

Beans, Beans the Magical Brain Fruit

Beans could just be the most underrated food in our diets. Most types of beans have high levels of vitamin B6 and folate, both of which help to lessen levels of homocysteine in the body. High homocysteine levels often indicate an increased risk of heart disease, stroke, and accelerated aging. Some of the beans that are high in vitamin B6 and folate include kidney beans, black beans, lima beans, and most other types of legumes.

Beans are usually high in the B-vitamin thiamine, which is integral to energy production and brain cell and cognitive function. Thiamine is needed to make an important brain messenger substance called acetylcholine, which therefore means that thiamine is imperative to healthy memory functioning.[35]

Kidney beans are high in the mineral manganese, which is needed to make an important enzyme in the body called "superoxide dismutase," or SOD. SOD disarms free radicals produced in the energy centres of the cells, thereby improving energy production and lessening oxidative damage in the body. A cup of kidney beans supplies your body with almost one-quarter of the daily recommended dose of manganese. Other good food sources include eggs, brown rice, green vegetables, blueberries, ginger, nuts, bananas, olives, and avocados.

A Pit Stop on the Road to Brain Health

Fruits that contain pits are among the most concentrated in flavonoids, which are protective and healing for the brain. Such fruits include apricots, peaches, plums, and cherries. Make them a regular part of your diet. And, for those of you on low carb diets, yes, they contain plentiful amounts of fruit sugars, the most important source of energy for your brain. And it is possible to eat them and still maintain a healthy weight. Weight loss should never be at the expense of your long-term health. If you've eliminated these important fruits from your diet, now is the time to add them back in.

TOP TWENTY BRAIN SUPERFOODS

As you have just learned, there are many great brain Superfoods. As part of *The Brain Wash* Plan, I encourage people to strive to eat at least five of these brain Superfoods daily. You'll learn more about *The Brain Wash* Plan in chapter 8. But, to help you get started, here are the Top Twenty Brain Superfoods:

Almonds
Avocados
Green or Black Tea
Blueberries
Celery
Celery Seeds
Cherries
Cocoa (Organic, Unsweetened only)
Flax Seeds and Flax Oil
Ginger
Kidney Beans and Other Beans
Leafy Greens
Olives and Olive Oil
Onions and Garlic
Purple and Red Grapes
Raw Walnuts

Fresh Sage
Tomatoes
Turmeric
Wild Salmon and Other Fatty Coldwater Fish

SUPPLEMENTING WITH CRITICAL BRAIN NUTRIENTS

There are many powerful nutrients and nutritional supplements that can assist you with your quest to create or maintain a healthy brain. Some are ideal for regular supplementation on an ongoing basis, while others may be best used in the prevention or treatment of specific health concerns.

MY TOP FIVE SUPPLEMENT PICKS FOR JUST ABOUT EVERYONE

While there are many great nutritional supplements suited for brain health, some stand out as so incredibly effective and so beneficial to many different brain functions that almost anyone would benefit from their use on a daily basis. It can be difficult to know which supplements to choose for daily use without needing a suitcase to hold them all. To help you in your pursuit of brain health, I've selected my favourite supplements for ongoing use, to improve the overall health of your brain, prevent brain disease, or help your brain heal if you are already suffering from a brain disorder. My top supplement picks include alpha lipoic acid, coenzyme Q10, chlorella, Cellfood, and probiotics.

Alpha lipoic acid

A potent antioxidant, alpha lipoic acid offers tremendous help in treating existing brain disease and in preventing the build up of free radicals in the brain—a major contributing factor in most brain diseases. Perhaps part of alpha lipoic acid's tremendous power is its ability to readily cross the blood-brain barrier, in addition to its potent free radical scavenging capacity.[36] As if that weren't enough, alpha lipoic acid gives a helping hand to other brain antioxidants like vitamins C and E and glutathione.[37] Everyone needs antioxidant support to protect brain health and ward off the symptoms typically associated with aging—is there anyone who's not aging?

Coenzyme Q10

A study presented at the annual meeting of the American Neurological Association in New York City suggests that the nutritional supplement coenzyme Q10 (CoQ10) could slow the progression of Parkinson's disease. Lead researcher Professor Clifford Shults of the University of California in San Diego and his colleagues enrolled eighty early-stage, non-levodopa-taking Parkinson's patients for the trial. The patients were randomly assigned treatment with three hundred, six hundred or twelve hundred milligrams per day of the nutrient coenzyme Q10 or a placebo. After eight months, patients who received the highest dose of CoQ10 fared significantly better than those who received the placebo. These highest dose patients had a forty-four percent reduction in disease progression, compared to the placebo group. Even patients taking only three hundred milligrams per day of CoQ10 were better able to carry out simple daily activities like dressing and washing and demonstrated better mental functioning and mood. Shults stresses that his study was small and therefore not conclusive, however it does suggest that CoQ10 may slow the progression of neurodegenerative diseases like Parkinson's.[38]

Earlier research provides evidence that the mitochondria, also known as the powerhouses of the body's cells, are impaired in Parkinson's patients.[39] Research also shows that CoQ10 is essential for proper energy production of these powerhouses in the cells.

Alzheimer's has been linked to mutations in the mitochondria of the DNA. Researchers found variations of a specific DNA mutation in the brains of sixty-five percent of people with Alzheimer's disease and none of the others.[40] While it is unclear whether the mutation is a contributing cause or an effect of the disease, attempting to ensure healthy functioning mitochondria is essential to great brain health. CoQ10 can power up every cell in your body and brain. CoQ10's overall capacity as a brain rejuvenator means it makes the cut as one of the top brain supplements for just about everyone.

Chlorella

Chlorella is truly deserving of the title "Brain Superfood" because of the many effects it has, both directly and indirectly, on improving brain health. Chlorella helps to remove heavy metals and pesticides from the body; it improves digestion and lessens constipation (you learned about the gut-brain connection in chapter 5); chlorella assists with mental concentration and focus, balances the blood by lowering acidity; and delivers tremendous nutritional value in the form of vitamins, minerals, and enzymes.

Chlorella is a type of algae that is superior in chlorophyll-content than other green food supplements like spirulina, blue-green algae, wheat grass, and barley grass. Chlorophyll is the green colour in plants that helps the body build healthy blood cells. Additionally, chlorella contains tough cell walls that give it a superior ability to eliminate toxins, heavy metals, and pesticides from the body.

European, Japanese, and American studies indicate chlorella's impressive success at strengthening the body's immune system while breaking down toxins, called "persistent hydrocarbons and metals," including DDT, PCBs, mercury, cadmium, and lead.[41]

As Dr. Joseph Mercola, MD, suggests, it will take at least three to six months of taking three grams daily for enough chlorella to build up in the body to start detoxifying heavy metals and other chemical toxins from your body. He also indicates that after the body's toxic burden of mercury is lowered from the intestines, it more readily migrates from other bodily tissues into the intestines, where it binds with chlorella to be removed in the stool.

Research also indicates that supplementing with chlorella helps the beneficial bacteria in your intestines, like lactobacillus, multiply at four times the normal rate, thereby greatly assisting with lessening infection, candida-overgrowth, and toxins in the bowels.

Because chlorella more closely resembles a food than a nutritional supplement, it is perishable. Purchase chlorella in an airtight container and keep it at cool temperatures away from oxygen for maximum potency.

Chlorella truly is a Superfood as well as a super supplement. Just about everyone would benefit from supplementing with chlorella.

Cellfood

Cellfood is a natural, liquid oxygen and nutritional supplement containing over one hundred minerals, amino acids, and enzymes. Cellfood delivers oxygen to the blood, where it can easily be carried to the brain. Unlike other oxygen supplements, which may flood the body with excessive oxygen at one time and insufficient amounts at other times, Cellfood appears to deliver oxygen as the body is able to use it. Cellfood also delivers valuable nutrients and enzymes alongside the oxygen to the body, thereby speeding detoxification and nourishing cells.

Recent studies by Iorio, Bianchi, and Storti, testing Cellfood's Biological Antioxidant Potential (BAP) found that it measured 64,747, which is tremendously high antioxidant potential. By comparison, it showed over thirty times more antioxidant capacity than blood.

While I am not a fan of naming specific product brands, occasionally a product is so impressive that it warrants such discussion. I've included more information about Cellfood in the resource section. Cellfood's impressive antioxidant power and broad spectrum nutrient and oxygen delivery make this one of my top picks for regular, ongoing supplementation for just about everyone.

Probiotics

You learned about probiotics and their role in preventing and treating brain disease in chapter 5. The ideal probiotic supplement includes lactobacillus acidophilus, lactobacillus bulgaricus, lactobacillus plantarum and bifidobacteria, especially bifidobacteria bifidum. The dose varies from product to product. Because probiotics play such an important role in brain health (and overall health) and are so commonly deficient, I recommend supplementing with them on a regular, ongoing basis.

MORE BRAIN BOOSTING SUPPLEMENTS

Boost Your Body's Glutathione Production

Glutathione, while available in many health food stores as a supplement, has shown that it is not usable to the body when taken directly in capsule or tablet form. However, this powerful antioxidant nutrient is made by the body, and research demonstrates that supplementation with the nutrient N-acetyl cysteine (NAC) and vitamin C, assists the body in increasing its own glutathione stores. Glutathione is an important nutrient in the detoxification process of many harmful chemicals, including neurotoxins, in the body. Glutathione also helps lessen free radicals linked to aging and most brain diseases.

POWER UP THE CELL'S POWER CENTRES

You learned about CoQ10's impressive rejuvenating abilities. There are other nutrients that power up the cell's power centres to ensure your brain has energy for all its functions. In many brain diseases the mitochondria are found to be impaired, limiting cellular ability to revitalize brain tissue. In addition to CoQ10, some of the other best brain supplements include the herb ginkgo biloba, which I will discuss in greater detail in the next chapter, the nutrients phosphatidylserine (PS), acetyl-L-carnitine, and NADH. All of these supplements have been extensively studied and reported on in many scientific journals. They show positive and proven results in helping to rejuvenate the mitochondria.[42]

Acetyl-L-Carnitine

The nutrient, acetyl-L-carnitine, is a modified version of an amino acid found in protein. Acetyl-L-carnitine is potent in assisting the creation of energy in brain cells by delivering essential fatty acids to them, and by assisting with brain cells' elimination of waste products. This nutrient is readily absorbed across the blood-brain barrier and is helpful in the manufacture of the brain messenger chemical acetylcholine. It has proven therapeutic for ALS at a dose of four hundred milligrams daily. Higher doses of one thousand milligrams three times per day helps with memory and communication between brain cells in Alzheimer's disease and has even been effective at delaying the progression of early-stage Alzheimer's disease.[43]

SAMe (S-Adenosylmethionine)

SAMe is a substance that occurs naturally in the body and enables many different biochemical processes to function properly. It is helpful in the treatment of depression. Four hundred to twelve hundred milligrams a day of SAMe appears to boost levels of well being and happiness by balancing neurotransmitter levels in the brain.[44] Avoid taking SAMe if you have bipolar disorder. If you are taking anti-depressant drugs you should consult a physician prior to, and during, supplementation with SAMe.

5-HTP

Low levels of the neurotransmitter serotonin are linked with depression and other mood regulation disorders, which you'll learn more about in the next chapter. While you can't take a serotonin pill to boost levels, you can help your body manufacture more by supplementing with 5-HTP and the herb St. John's wort (more on this herb in the next chapter as well).

5-HTP stands for 5-hydroxytryptophan, one of the raw materials needed to manufacture adequate serotonin levels. The success of 5-HTP in treating conditions like depression that are linked to low serotonin levels has been extensively documented.

The standard dose for depression is fifty milligrams three times daily. If symptoms have not improved after two weeks, increase the dosage to one hundred milligrams three times daily. Occasionally nausea is a symptom of taking 5-HTP, but gradually increasing the dose in this manner helps to lessen any possibility of nausea. Enteric-coated capsules or tablets are also helpful to lessen the risk of nausea. You can also take the supplement with food. While not necessarily suitable for everyone, 5-HTP does have an important role in the treatment of mood regulation disorders or for those times in life when we may be more susceptible to these disorders.

Pectin

Pectin is a specific type of fibre usually extracted from apples or citrus fruit. As a supplement, it may be found under the name "modified citrus pectin." Pectin binds to heavy metals in the bloodstream, thereby helping the liver to flush them out of the body through the intestines, according to Nan Kathryn Fuchs, PhD, a nutrition researcher.[45] Based on research from California's Amitabha Medical Center, five grams of pectin daily is enough to flush almost seventy percent of heavy metals out of most people's bodies within months. Foods high in pectin include apples, bananas, beets, cabbage, carrots, citrus fruits, dried peas, and okra. You'll learn more about pectin and using it as part of a heavy metal detox in chapter 10.

TOP BRAIN BOOSTING NUTRIENTS

5-HTP
Alpha Lipoic Acid
B12
B6
B-vitamins Complex
Blueberry Extract
Cellfood
Cherry Extract
Chlorella
Coenzyme Q10
Folate (B9)
Ginger
Ginkgo Biloba
Grape Extract
Acetyl-L-Carnitine
Magnesium
Multimineral Containing Iron, Selenium, and Zinc
N-Acetyl Cysteine
NADH
Niacin (B3)
Pectin
Phosphatidylserine (PS)
Probiotics

Resveratrol
Sage
Turmeric
Vitamin E

DETOXIFY THE YEARS AWAY

Since toxins damage cells, and this damage is linked with premature aging, it is imperative to lessen the toxic load of your organ systems by reducing your exposure to harmful substances such as pharmaceutical drugs, alcohol, sugar, cigarette smoke, coffee, chemical food additives, and trans fats and rancid fats found in fried, processed, and over-heated foods.

Due to the damaging role that toxins play in our bodies, it is not surprising that regularly engaging in a cleansing program can protect cells from damage and even help to reverse cellular damage. The National Institute on Aging found that detoxification increases a person's lifespan as well or better than caloric restriction, a common strategy to slow the effects of aging.

Depending on the source of the toxins in your body, your approach to detoxification may be different than someone else's. When it comes to purifying your body, there really isn't a good "one size fits all" type of program. You may need to eliminate candida if you have a fungal overgrowth, or your focus may be better served in eliminating heavy metals from your body, or both.

Nutrients Required for Detoxification

Detoxifying is the process of assisting your body in its ability to eliminate harmful toxic build-up by improving the function of your many detox organs, including the intestines, kidneys, bladder, lymphatic system, liver, gall bladder, respiratory system, skin, and blood. Unlike fasting, in which you eliminate food and drink only water, a good detoxification plan should include adequate amounts of healthy foods to ensure you have all the nutrients required to detoxify properly.

It is imperative to ensure that you consume the nutrients your body requires for proper detoxification and to ensure a healthy brain.

Vitamins	Some of the Best Food Sources
Beta carotene	Carrots, beets, leafy greens, melon, squash, yams
Folic Acid	Mushrooms, nuts, whole grains, broccoli, asparagus, beans, lettuce, spinach, beet greens, sweet potatoes, leafy greens
Niacin	Avocados, dates, figs, green vegetables, whole grains, brown rice, sunflower seeds
Panthothenic Acid	Green vegetables, peas, beans, kale, cauliflower, sweet potatoes, whole grains, brown rice
Riboflavin	Whole grains, almonds, sunflower seeds, currants, asparagus, broccoli, leafy greens
Vitamin B1 (Thiamine)	Brown rice, nuts, seeds, nut butters, oats, asparagus, beets, leafy greens, plums, raisins
Vitamin B12	Kelp, bananas, peanuts, concord grapes, sprouts
Vitamin B6 (Pyridoxine)	Bananas, avocados, whole grains, cantaloupe, walnuts, soybeans, peanuts, pecans, leafy greens, green peppers, carrots
Vitamin C	Citrus fruits, apples, strawberries, beet greens, spinach, cabbage, broccoli, cauliflower, kale, tomatoes, sweet potatoes, peppers, papaya, swiss chard, squash
Vitamin E	Whole grains, brussel sprouts, leafy greens, spinach, cold-pressed vegetable oils, soybeans, brown rice

Minerals	Some of the Best Food Sources
Calcium	Leafy greens, tofu, soy beans, soy milk, almonds, carob, sesame seeds, tahini, navy beans, walnuts, millet, kelp, carrot juice, oats, broccoli
Copper	Almonds, peanuts, dried peas and beans, avocados, plums, cherries, citrus fruits, raisins, whole-grains, oats, leafy greens
Germanium	Garlic, shiitake mushrooms, onions, whole-grains
Iron	Apricots, peaches, bananas, raisins, figs, whole rye, walnuts, kelp, dry beans, leafy greens, asparagus, potatoes
Manganese	Nuts, whole grains, spinach, beets, beet greens, brussels sprouts, peas, kelp, tea, apricots, blueberries, bananas, citrus fruits
Molybdenum	Brown rice, millet, buckwheat, legumes, leafy greens, whole-grains
Selenium	Brown rice, soy beans, Brazil nuts, kelp, garlic, mushrooms, pineapple, onions, tomatoes, broccoli
Sulphur	Radish, turnip, onions, celery, horseradish, kale, soybeans, cucumber
Zinc	Sprouted seeds, pumpkin seeds, sunflower seeds, onions, nuts, leafy greens, peas, beets, beet greens

Anti-Candida/Anti-Bacterial Cleansing Diet

If you suspect you may have an overgrowth of harmful candida albicans in your intestines, following an anti-candida diet may be helpful to restore beneficial bacteria. Here are some of the most important considerations in cleansing your intestinal tract of candida, other fungi, and bacteria.

Refrain from eating sugar, foods with yeast, and alcohol. That includes all sweets, breads made with yeast, and alcoholic beverages, especially wine and beer. Also, avoid dairy products (especially cheeses). Refrain from eating foods that typically have moulds or yeasts present on them, including peanuts and all types of vinegar except apple cider vinegar. Apple cider vinegar actually helps kill candida bacteria.

Eat plenty of fruits and vegetables, both steamed and raw. Eat some high-protein foods at each meal. That includes beans and legumes, soy milk, organic eggs, and tofu. Eat foods such as garlic, onions, scallions, and horseradish, all of which destroy harmful yeasts and parasites. Season your food with herbs that have similar effects, including basil, dill, oregano, and ginger.

Choose anti-parasitic herbs from those mentioned in the following chapter to help lessen candida overgrowth in the intestines.

The same diet will have beneficial effects on balancing beneficial flora and will help kill harmful bacteria in the intestines.

In addition to some of the direct brain benefits of magnesium mentioned earlier, it is one of nature's best natural and gentle laxatives. It adds water to the stool to assist with its easy elimination from the body. Eat foods that are high in magnesium, such as apples, figs, peaches, kale, chard, celery, beet greens, brown rice, sesame seeds, sunflower seeds, almonds, and soybeans. In addition, supplement your diet with four hundred milligrams of magnesium per day.

Liver Detoxifying

Regularly detoxifying your liver is essential to overall brain health. As you learned earlier in this book, the liver has the enormous job of neutralizing and assisting with elimination of the onslaught of toxins our bodies are exposed to. Liver detoxification helps to ensure your liver has the nutritional and herbal support it needs to effectively handle this job, thereby lessening the number of toxins that will circulate in your bloodstream or brain.

Eat lots of garlic, onions, and broccoli since these foods contain sulphur that is required to increase enzyme activity (and therefore increase liver-cleansing activity).

TOP TWELVE LIVER SUPPORTING FOODS

Oatmeal
This complex carbohydrate (the good kind) is slow to digest and helps to keep blood sugar levels stable while keeping you feeling full. Research also shows that consuming oatmeal reduces a person's cravings for fatty foods. Be sure to eat the unsweetened kind.

Leafy Greens
Spinach, spring mix, mustard greens, and other dark leafy greens are good sources of fibre and powerhouses of nutrition. Research demonstrates that leafy greens' high concentration of vitamins and antioxidants helps prevent hunger while protecting you from heart disease, cancer, cataracts, and memory loss.

Olives and Olive Oil
Being rich in healthy fats, olives and olive oil help to reduce cravings for junky foods and keep you feeling full. Research shows that the monounsaturated fats that are plentiful in these foods help reduce high blood pressure.

Beans and Legumes
Legumes are the best source of fibre of any foods. They help to stabilize blood sugar while keeping you regular. They are also high in potassium, a critical mineral that reduces dehydration and the risk of high blood pressure and stroke. One legume, soy, is particularly good

for burning fat. Isoflavones found in soy foods speed the breakdown of stored fat. In one study, those who consumed high amounts of soy products shed three times more superfluous weight than did their counterparts who ate no soy.

Garlic and Onions
These yummy foods contain phytochemicals that break down fatty deposits in the body, while also breaking down cholesterol, killing viruses, bacteria, and fungi, and protecting against heart disease.

Tomatoes
Packed with vitamin C and lycopene, tomatoes stimulate the production of the amino acid known as carnitine. Carnitine helps speed the body's fat-burning capacity by one-third. Lycopene is a powerful antioxidant that cuts the risk of heart disease by twenty-nine percent.

Nuts
Raw, unsalted nuts provide your body with essential fatty acids that help burn fat. Their high nutrient content also lowers the risk of heart attack by sixty percent. Research shows that consuming nuts can be as effective as cholesterol-lowering drugs to reduce high cholesterol levels, not to mention they taste better and have no nasty side effects.[46]

Cayenne
This hot spice lessens the risk of excess insulin in the body, by speeding metabolism and lowering blood sugar levels, before the excess insulin can result in fat stores.[47]

Turmeric
The popular spice used primarily in Indian cooking, contains the highest known source of beta carotene, the antioxidant that helps protect the liver from free radical damage. Turmeric also helps your liver heal (see below) while it assists your body to metabolise fats by decreasing the fat storage rate in liver cells.[48]

Cinnamon

Researchers at the United States Department of Agriculture showed that one teaspoon of cinnamon with food helps metabolise sugar up to twenty times better.[49] Excess sugar in the blood can lead to fat storage.

Flaxseeds and Flaxseed Oil

Flaxseeds and flaxseed oil attract oil-soluble toxins that are lodged in the fatty tissues of the body to escort them out.[50]

Nutrients for Improving Liver Function

Take one or two digestive enzyme tablets with every meal. Ideally, the digestive enzyme you take should include proteases I, II, and III, maltase, amylase, lipase, cellulase, peptidase, lactase, and invertase.

For optimal liver cleansing, take two tablespoons of high quality, cold-pressed flaxseed oil as part of your diet. In addition, add one to two tablespoons of freshly ground flaxseeds (use a small coffee grinder), sprinkled on food, after it has been cooked. Avoid cooking flaxseeds or flaxseed oil.

Eat plenty of garlic and onions since they are high in sulphur, which is important to help your liver function optimally. In addition, eat plenty of the other top liver supporting foods mentioned above.

Lecithin helps the liver metabolise fats and reduce cholesterol. It contains a substance called phosphatidylcholine and essential fatty acids that help keep liver cells healthy and help prevent fatty deposits from building up in the liver. Lecithin also helps reduce high blood pressure by allowing the blood vessels to relax to allow better blood flow. You can get lecithin in soy foods like soy milk, tofu, and miso, as well as in organic eggs. Alternatively, take four thousand milligrams of lecithin in capsule form daily.

BUILDING A BETTER BABY BRAIN

Okay, now you know all about the most powerful brain supporting nutrients and supplements available from nature, and how to support your body's most important systems for optimal brain health. But what about the needs of growing brains? A mother's diet is not only her growing baby's diet; what a mother ingests and assimilates forms the very cells of her growing fetus. You learned earlier that the most critical period of brain development is during pregnancy until the end of the third year of life. If a period of malnutrition occurs anytime during those years, it is possible that irreversible brain damage can occur.

Carol Simontacci, certified clinical nutritionist and author of the book *The Crazy Makers: How the Food Industry is Destroying Our Brains and Harming Our Children*, describes the importance of nutrition on a fetus' brain development: "When a mother consumes a diet that undersupplies fats, proteins, carbohydrates, vitamins, minerals, and water for both her and her baby, some part of the baby's brain development will be curtailed. Some structure will go unbuilt; some function will not be performed."[51]

During pregnancy, large amounts of healthy fats are theoretically deposited into the brain tissue from Omega-3, Omega-6, and other fatty acids. I say "theoretically" because the growing child can't deposit what isn't present. So, if the mother's diet is deficient in any of these essential fatty acids, which most women's are, then the baby's brain will not develop properly.

Four of the primary minerals needed for optimum brain development include calcium, potassium, zinc, and magnesium. They serve many functions. They activate hundreds of brain enzymes; manufacture energy at the cellular level; transfer nerve signals; regulate enzyme functions; increase the passage of nutrients in and out of brain cells; maintain acid-alkaline balance throughout the brain; eliminate toxic by-products of metabolism; ensure proper cellular replication in DNA; strengthen cellular membranes; and regulate sugar flow to the brain for fuel.[52] Yet, most people don't get enough of these nutrients to maintain their own health, let alone to support a developing fetus in the womb or infant through breastfeeding.

So, you may be thinking, "Yes, but isn't infant formula full of all the essential nutrients needed for a child's brain development?" The answer is "not even close." Some people even wrongly assume that infant formula is superior to breast milk. That's a frightening misperception that is harming our children's brain development.

If a woman is eating a healthy diet, her breast milk will contain friendly bacteria, immunoglobulins, enzymes that destroy harmful bacteria and aid digestibility of the milk, growth factors, hormones, non-essential amino acids, healthy fatty acids, essential amino acids, vitamins, and minerals. Infant formula contains none of the former ingredients and only subpar amounts of the latter four ingredients. Some infant formula doesn't even contain healthy fatty acids, meaning it comprises only a handful of vitamins, minerals, and essential amino acids. According to Simontacci's research, there are approximately one hundred elements found in breast milk that are missing from infant formula. She adds, "The absence of any of these biofactors has the potential for long-term damage to the vulnerable child."[53]

Infant formulas vary in mineral content by as much as five hundred percent. Formulas routinely provide excessive amounts of some amino acids that block the uptake of other, essential amino acids like tryptophan, which assists with the manufacture of serotonin, a calming neurotransmitter that helps lessen aggression, anxiety, depression, and the likelihood of other brain disorders.[54]

Simontacci emphasizes the significance of this research: "When infants are fed synthetic formula instead of breast milk, they have less of the important brain-modelling DHA and other Omega-3 fatty acids and arachidonic acids in their blood, thereby making them susceptible to a form of brain damage—the building blocks for brain material are missing."[55]

Breastfeeding poses difficulties for some women. A host of problems can occur, and the most common response of medical doctors is to suggest bottle-feeding. This is unfortunate not only because of the subpar nutrients in formula, but also because the vast majority of breastfeeding difficulties can be quickly resolved through natural therapies, especially through herbal remedies. This is one area in which nature's medicines vastly and irrefutably out-perform medical science's ability to help; yet, most women have no idea that support is available to them. Work with a medical herbalist or doctor of natural medicine to help find the natural remedies that will be best for your specific situation.

The good news is that for most women, breastfeeding can provide their babies with exactly what is needed for optimal development. Taking care of yourself is taking care of your baby's future, too.

c h a p t e r
7

Healing Herbs

"Don't dig your grave with your own knife and fork."
~ English Proverb

▧ ▧ ▧ ▧ ▧ ▧ ▧

In chapter 7, "Healing Herbs" you will learn

- the best herbs that directly influence the brain;
- the herbs that work on the digestive tract, which, as you learned in Chapter 5, is impera- tive to healthy brain functioning; and
- homeopathic remedies for detoxifying brain damag- ing alcohol, drugs, vaccines, and more from the body.

▧ ▧ ▧ ▧ ▧ ▧ ▧

Many people discount herbs in the prevention and treatment of brain diseases, believing them to be ineffective or only mildly effective. Pharmaceutical companies with billion-dollar advertising budgets have attempted to brainwash us into thinking that only drugs are helpful in the treatment of such serious disorders. And, of course, they encourage the belief that this "potent medicine" comes at a high financial price and that nasty side effects are a small price to pay for results.

But the reality couldn't be further from the truth. While Mother Nature's medicines humbly lay upon the earth in her rainforests, wilderness, and jungles devoid of any loud-mouthed marketing man- agers or slick advertising campaigns, they show tremendous promise in the prevention and treatment of brain disease.

The pharmaceutical giants won't tell you that Mother Nature is the genius behind their success and that her botanical medicines form the basis for over seventy percent of their medicines. However, in the hands of these multinational corporations, these potent botanical medicines with few side effects have been depleted and denatured until they are reduced to their active ingredients, which are then synthesized in the name of profit-making patents. After all, you can't patent herbs that have existed for many thousands of years. And without a patent, profits drop drastically. (For a look at the ethical and business side of patents, I recommend reading the eye-opening book *Patents, Profits and Power*.) But once the active ingredients of an herb are synthesized to form medicines, the harmful health effects escalate as quickly as the corporate profits.

There are hundreds of herbs that have been scientifically validated for their effectiveness against as many diseases, and which have stood the test of time over many thousands of years in humankind's history. While many warrant discussion, due to space considerations I've selected only a handful of some of the most effective herbs against brain diseases and the inflammation that is often linked to these disorders. Some of these potent herbs include sage, turmeric, periwinkle, ginkgo biloba, oregano, rosemary, parsley, ginger, St. John's wort, kava, and rhodiola. Because herbs are potent medicine, it is important to consult with your doctor before you start taking any herbs to prevent drug-herb interactions.

A WISE SAGE

In Germany's popular Commission E monographs, sage is recommended primarily for dyspepsia, excessive perspiration, and inflammation of the mouth and nose, and it is now being considered as a potential treatment for Alzheimer's disease. The German Commission E monographs comprise some of the most comprehensive information on the safety and efficacy of herbs and phytomedicines, The Commission was established by the German Minister of Health almost three decades ago and its monographs recognize many herbs as medicine.

British researchers followed up on four-century-old writings of renowned herbalists John Gerard and Nicholas Culpepper. In 1597, John Gerard wrote that sage "is singularly good for the head and brain and quickeneth the nerves and memory." In 1652, Nicholas Culpepper wrote that sage "also heals the memory, warming and quickening the senses." Nicola Tildesley and his colleagues opted to test the truth of these claims by conducting a study of sage's therapeutic properties on a group of forty-four adults between the ages of eighteen and thirty-seven. Some participants were given capsules of sage oil while others were given a placebo of sunflower oil. Results showed that those who took the sage oil performed significantly better at memory tests than those who took the placebo.[1]

A number of significant effects on cognition were noted with the sage species *salvia lavandulifolia*. The effects included improvements in both immediate and delayed word recall scores. The researchers concluded that sage oil is capable of affecting mood and cognition in healthy young adults.[2]

Research by the same team showed that sage inhibits acetylcholinesterase (AChE). AChE breaks down the neurotransmitter acetylcholine, which plays an important role in memory and is depleted in patients with Alzheimer's disease.[3]

Researchers hope that their findings may translate into an effective natural treatment for Alzheimer's. As a result sage is being tested as a potential treatment for Alzheimer's disease.

There are several species of sage, including *salvia miltiorrhiza*—a commonly used ingredient in Chinese medicines, known as "dan shen"; *salvia divinorum*—found in Mexico and has a reputation as a hallucinogen; *salvia officinalis*—the most commonly used type of sage in Western European medicine; and *salvia lavandulifolia*—which is Spanish sage.

Additional research suggests that one or more constituents of *salvia lavandulifolia*, when taken orally, crosses the gastrointestinal and blood-brain barriers to reach the brain and may inhibit a potentially brain damaging substance, called "cholinesterase" in select brain areas.[4] Since sage oil is a very low-risk natural medicine, it may be used by people concerned about memory or by those already suffering from memory disorders.

THE CURRY FACTOR

Turmeric (*curcuma longa*) is the yellowish spice commonly used in Indian food. Turmeric's main therapeutic ingredient is called "curcumin" and has been shown to deplete nerve endings of substance P, a pain neurotransmitter. Research shows that *curcumin* suppresses pain, without the harmful side effects of pharmaceutical drugs, making turmeric effective for relief of pain linked to neurological disorders.

Other studies by Greg Cole, PhD, associate director of the Alzheimer's Disease Research Center at the University of California in Los Angeles, show that the yellow pigment in turmeric, curcumin, is both an inflammation- and amyloid plaque-fighter.[5] Still further research conducted by a medical team at a graduate school at Kanazawa University demonstrated that curcumin prevents the development of a substance called amyloid beta (AB) in the brain.[6] This substance is linked as a causative factor for Alzheimer's disease.

Early evidence of the link between inflammation and Alzheimer's disease started when researchers Patrick McGeer at the University of British Columbia and Joe Rogers of Sun Health Research Center in Arizona, sifted through a decade of hospital drug records and found that arthritis patients who were regularly treated with strong anti-inflammatory drugs were seven times less likely to develop Alzheimer's. Seven times![7] Since then researchers have been looking for effective natural medicines against inflammation for the natural treatment of Alzheimer's disease, and that is where turmeric really shines.

Recent findings indicate that ingesting twelve hundred milligrams of *curcumin* had the same effect as taking three hundred milligrams of the anti-inflammatory drug phenylbutazone.[8]

While it is hard to know how much curcumin is present in the powdered spice form of turmeric, it is still a valuable way to ingest this important herb. It is safe to take up to four tablespoons of turmeric mixed into water or honey and water per day. I find the honey-turmeric-water mixture to be far more palatable than taking turmeric in water or juice. Go easy on the honey though, or you'll risk flooding your brain with excessive sugars. For ease, turmeric can also be ingested in capsule form. In that case, choose a standardized extract with fifteen hundred milligrams of *curcumin* content per day (look for extracts called *cucuma longa* 17,8; xanthorrizol from curcuma xanthorrhiza Roxh11; and beta-turmerone from curcuma zedoaria Roscoe11).

PERIWINKLE: THE BLUE FLOWER FOR GREY MATTER

Periwinkle is a European plant used by herbalists to treat nervous disorders, epilepsy, hysteria, and nightmares. Research shows that vinpocetine, a derivative of vincamine, a natural compound in periwinkle, helps transport oxygen and glucose to the brain. Since the brain needs both to function optimally, periwinkle may be beneficial against brain disease. Vinpocetine is a vasodilator and cerebral metabolic enhancer, meaning it gives the brain all it needs of both oxygen and glucose.[9]

With around one hundred studies conducted on vinpocetine's effects on humans, mostly in Hungary, it is not surprising that it has been used by Hungarian doctors to treat senility and blood vessel disorders in the brain for twenty-five years. In these studies it appears to boost memory and cognition in healthy people and in those with mild to moderate forms of dementia.

A double-blind study in 1985 in the *European Journal of Clinical Pharmacology*, researchers tested vinpocetine's effect on the short-term memory of twelve healthy women. The women who took forty milligrams of vinpocetine three times per day for two days scored thirty percent higher on short-term memory tests than the women in the placebo group.[10]

In another double-blind study in 1991, published in *International Clinical Psychopharmacology*, researchers tested 165 people with mild to moderate dementia. After sixteen weeks, twenty-one percent of those taking thirty to sixty milligrams of vinpocetine daily reported a decline in symptom severity, compared to only seven percent of those taking the placebo.[11]

Vinpocetine is a powerful free radical scavenger. Used regularly, periwinkle, or its active ingredient, vinpocetine, may help to prevent senility and dementia, by preventing damage to the blood vessels in the brain caused by free radicals. Vinpocetine also thins blood, boosts circulation in your brain, and improves the brain's ability to absorb nutrients, all of which improve brain function.[12] Research shows that vinpocetine works as well as ginkgo biloba—an herbal superstar for aiding brain oxygenation—in improving memory and cognitive abilities.[13]

Periwinkle and vinpocetine are showing tremendous promise as a therapy for many brain diseases, especially stroke recovery. It is used throughout Europe and Japan as a natural therapy for stroke since it helps increase blood flow to areas of the brain with minimal function.[14]

Experts typically suggest dosages of up to ten milligrams daily, taken with food. Up to forty-five milligrams is considered a safe daily dose; but, doses above ten milligrams should be supervised by a health care practitioner. Vinpocetine appears to be safe for short- or long-term use. The effects tend to be fast-acting, not cumulative. In rare cases, someone may experience minor stomach upset and a dry mouth. Check with your doctor before taking either vinpocetine or periwinkle, especially if you are taking blood-thinning medications.

GINKGO BILOBA

Dr. Michael Murray, author of *Dr. Murray's Total Body Tune-Up*, describes the many beneficial uses of ginkgo biloba, including assisting to ease "cerebral vascular insufficiency (insufficient blood flow to the brain), dementia, depression, impotence, inner ear dysfunction (vertigo, tinnitus, etc.), multiple sclerosis, neuralgia and neuropathy, peripheral vascular insufficiency (intermittent claudication, Raynaud's syndrome, etc.), premenstrual syndrome, retinopathy (macular degeneration, diabetic retinopathy, etc.), and vascular fragility."[15]

Ginkgo is an herb found to be especially helpful with early-stage Alzheimer's disease. In Germany, ginkgo is approved as a treatment for Alzheimer's. A study of forty patients with early-stage Alzheimer's disease, showed that 240 milligrams of ginkgo biloba extract taken daily for three months produced noticeable improvements in memory, mood, and attention.[16] Since then numerous other studies have shown similar positive effects on early-stage Alzheimer's disease.

Opt for ginkgo biloba standardized extract that contains twenty-four percent ginkgoflavonglycosides, also called "flavone glycosides," the active ingredient which has the capacity to increase blood flow to the brain and lessen symptoms like depression, memory loss, and dizziness, all of which can be the result of reduced blood flow to the brain.

Ginkgo also helps improve the availability of energy to brain cells. With more energy, the brain is more capable of metabolising its fuel—glucose. Ginkgo also appears to be an effective antioxidant that prevents free radical damage. It is such a beneficial herb that it is highly advisable to take for its many anti-aging effects. For ginkgo's preventive effects, forty milligrams three times a day is ideal. For brain diseases, the dose should be increased to eighty milligrams three times a day.

OREGACYN P73

Dr. Cass Ingram reported on a clinical pilot trial conducted on patients diagnosed with amyotrophic lateral sclerosis (ALS) to assess the benefits of a natural herbal product called Oregacyn P73—a proprietary blend of wild spice oils, including oregano, cumin and sage, combined with oregano juice. These patients had varying degrees of symptom and disease progression. Amyotrophic lateral sclerosis, also known as Lou Gehrig's disease, is a neuromuscular condition characterized by weakness, muscle wasting, and increased reflexes. It involves degeneration of motor neurons, killing fifty percent of patients within only eighteen months of diagnosis. Only ten percent of people with ALS live more than ten years.

The study involved eighteen patients from Canada and the United States and divided patients into three groups: patients in group A were given Oregacyn P73, one capsule, twice daily; those in group B were given oregano juice, one tablespoon, twice daily; and group C were given both Oregacyn P73 and oregano juice in the same dose as the other groups. Treatment was continued for ninety to 120 days. The researchers attempted to determine whether the antiseptic properties and antioxidant activities of oregano juice and the spice oils found in Oregacyn P73 had any effect on symptoms associated with ALS.

Thirty-nine percent of the participants reported an improvement in their symptoms at the end of the study. Thirty-three percent reported their symptoms as the same as prior to starting the study, and twenty-eight percent reported a worsening of symptoms linked with disease progression. Those who reported an improvement in their symptoms saw improvements in breathing, swelling, pain, and swallowing.

The study demonstrated the potential benefit of these spice oils and juice on symptoms of ALS. The author of the study indicates that it was intended as a pilot study only and that further study of this patient population using varied doses and longer duration may be beneficial in managing symptoms of ALS.[17] However, since there appear to be few and mild effects of taking these oils, it may be a good option for those already suffering from the disease, particularly in light of the disease prognosis using existing therapies.

Keep in mind that there are many types of oregano oil on the market, most of which use a different species than the one used in the above study. Long-term use of some of these other species can have potentially damaging effects on the liver. No negative liver effects have been noted in studies using P73, according to the manufacturers.

ROSEMARY

This pine-like herb does more than just spice up a roast of beef, it offers anti-inflammatory protection to the delicate human brain. Rosemary increases blood flow to the head and brain, thereby improving concentration.[18]

Historically, herbalists have used rosemary to strengthen memory. In England, rosemary's memory strengthening ability was translated to mean that it would improve fidelity. As a result it was often given as a gift for the bride or groom as part of their wedding ceremony. Perhaps the gift-giver thought the herb would help the newlywed remember his or her vows.

PARSLEY: MORE THAN A GARNISH

Perhaps you've tossed this herbal garnish aside in favour of delving further into your meal. If so, you may be missing out on one of the healthiest parts of the meal. Parsley is loaded with natural healing compounds that can help protect your brain. Ancient Greeks, on the other hand, regarded parsley as a sacred food, often adorning the winners of athletic contests with it.

It contains a substance called myristicin, which is a proven tumour inhibitor. It is considered a "chemoprotective" substance, meaning that it can help neutralize different types of carcinogens found in cigarette smoke, charred food, and the smoke created by trash incineration.[19]

Myristicin also activates an enzyme in the body called glutathione-S-transerase, which helps attach glutathione to substances that would otherwise do damage to the body. This process eliminates many toxic substances in the body before they can potentially cross the blood-brain barrier.

Parsley also contains a particularly healing group of nutrients called flavonoids, and one flavonoid in particular, called "luteolin." Luteolin is a potent antioxidant that combines with highly reactive molecules to prevent damage to cells. Since brain and nerve cells are particularly vulnerable to this type of damage, parsley is a great addition to everyone's diet.

Parsley also contains significant amounts of key nutrients, like vitamin C and vitamin A, both of which are antioxidants that protect the cells. Parsley contains folate, which is critical to keep the body's levels of a dangerous substance called homocysteine in check. Homocysteine levels are frequently used as a gauge for heart disease and stroke risk. It is imperative to lower levels of homocysteine when they are found to be high, and to keep these levels low throughout life. Folate is helpful in this process. You'll need to eat more parsley than just the garnish on your plate, however. A regular dose of the Middle Eastern salad, tabbouleh, which is made with plentiful amounts of parsley, might be a good start. You can also add parsley leaves to any fresh vegetable juice during the juicing process to gain the benefit of fresh parsley juice.

GINGERROOT

Not just great in stir-fries, ginger is one herb that can do more than add flavour and spice to just about any dish, it also exhibits antioxidant effects and the ability to lessen the formation of inflammation in the body. Ginger contains potent anti-inflammatory compounds called "gingerols" that work their magic on many types of inflammation in the body. A study in the November 2003 issue of *Life Sciences* indicates that ginger offers free radical protection through one of its many active constituents, called 6-gingerol. 6-gingerol has been shown to significantly inhibit the production of nitric oxide, a highly reactive nitrogen molecule that quickly forms a very damaging free radical called "peroxynitrite."[20]

Another study in the November 2003 issue of *Radiation Research* found that mice given ginger for five days prior to being exposed to radiation, not only avoided an increase in free radical damage to fats in the body, but also experienced a far smaller depletion of glutathione, one of the body's most important antioxidants.[21] Since the brain contains high levels of fats and is negatively impacted by radiation exposure and free radicals, ginger shows promise in protecting the brain.

According to Dr. Krishna C. Srivastava, ginger is superior to non-steroidal anti-inflammatory drugs (NSAIDs) in alleviating inflammation. This is important since physicians sometimes recommend anti-inflammatory drugs to treat brain disease linked to inflammation. Unlike NSAIDs that work on only one level of inflammation (blocking the substances that cause inflammation), ginger works on at least two mechanisms:

- Ginger blocks the formation of prostaglandins and leukotrienes, chemicals that are linked to the development of inflammation in the body; and

- Ginger also has antioxidant properties that actually break down inflammation and acidity in the body.

Ginger, eaten or used as a supplement on a regular basis, can have a protective effect by decreasing inflammation that occurs in the brain. One to ten grams per day of ginger root is an anti-inflammatory daily dose.

ST. JOHN'S WORT

St. John's wort (*hypericum perforatum*) is nature's Prozac, with a substantially better safety record. Its effectiveness for treating depression has been proven in dozens of double-bind studies, even in contrast to anti-depressant medications. This herb is at least as effective as drugs in the treatment of mild to moderate depression, without the long list of horrible side effects.

There has been some media hype over the use of St. John's wort, which is a bit misplaced. Most problems associated with the herb's use have been to do with drug interactions. People need to start recognizing that herbs are Mother Nature's medicines and they need to be treated with caution, especially when taken in combination with drugs manufactured by the pharmaceuticals. St. John's wort may interact with up to half of all drugs, either prescription or over-the-counter, so it is important to use caution while taking it, as you should with any medicine. However, St. John's wort's ability to interact with pharmaceutical drugs does not make it dangerous on its own, only with drug use. The drug manufacturers and media are quick to point the finger at St. John's wort, not the long list of drugs many people consume.

Currently St. John's wort is most effective against mild to somewhat severe depression. It is best to take a standardized extract of 0.3 percent hypericin, the active ingredient, at a dosage of nine hundred milligrams per day. If you are taking antidepressant medications like Prozac, Zoloft, Paxil, Effexor, or any other, you need to be closely monitored by your medical doctor, should you wish to use St. John's wort, to avoid what is known as "serotonin syndrome." On its own, there are no cases of St. John's wort causing serotonin syndrome, which is characterized by fever, shivering, sweating, diarrhea, muscle spasms, and confusion; but, serotonin syndrome is a possibility when combining the herb with drugs.

As I mentioned in chapter 1, serotonin is an important brain messenger, known as a neurotransmitter. Depression is typically the result of an improper balance of brain chemicals that regulate mood, particularly serotonin deficiency. Both St. John's wort and pharmaceutical drugs are intended to help the body increase serotonin in the brain, but, combined this mixture may over-stimulate production.

Some of the symptoms of low serotonin levels, as indicated by Dr. Murray, include "aggression, alcoholism, anxiety, attention deficit disorder, bulimia, carbohydrate cravings, chronic pain disorders (such as fibromyalgia), depression, epilepsy, headaches (migraines, tension headaches, chronic headaches), hyperactivity, insomnia, myoclonus (muscle twitching), obesity, obsessive-compulsive disorder, panic disorders, premenstrual syndrome, schizophrenia, seasonal affective disorder ("winter depression"), and suicidal thoughts and behaviour."[22]

Combined with the nutrient 5-HTP, that you learned about in the last chapter, St. John's wort can help treat virtually all conditions linked to low serotonin levels.

RHODIOLA ROSEA

An herb commonly prescribed in traditional Chinese medicine as an antioxidant, Rhodiola has been effective in the treatment of age-related disorders. One of a only a handful of herbs known as "adaptogens," which help the body cope with a variety of stressors, *rhodiola rosea* may be helpful for mild to moderate depression.

In one study, the active ingredient called salidroside, was effective at warding off damage caused by the excitotoxin glutamate. As you learned earlier, glutamate and its many derivatives, including monosodium glutamate are rampant in the food processing industry. This study shows promise in helping people to deal with unexpected glutamate exposures and the nervous system damage the toxin can cause.

Numerous studies conducted in Eastern Europe indicate that rhodiola improves cognitive function and reduces mental fatigue.[23]

Take one hundred to two hundred milligrams three times a day, standardized to three percent rosavin, another active ingredient in this powerful herb. Be aware that taking more than fifteen hundred milligrams per day can cause irritability or insomnia.

YOHIMBE

One study suggests that the herb yohimbe, used in traditional Indian Ayurvedic medicine, could dramatically reduce falls among Parkinson's patients. While only a small study of eleven people with Parkinson's, the study revealed that the herb slashed falls by fifty percent.[24] The research on yohimbe is still in its infancy but the herb shows promise to improve the motor decline linked with some brain diseases.

TOP HERBS FOR BRAIN HEALING

Gingerroot
Oregano
Parsley
Periwinkle
Rosemary
Sage
St. John's wort
Turmeric
Yohimbe

THE DIGESTION-CONNECTION

As you learned in the previous chapters, maintaining a healthy digestive tract is essential to brain health as well. Here are some of the best herbs to help eliminate candida and harmful bacterial overgrowth.

Many herbs promote intestinal cleansing and the elimination of toxins and built-up fecal matter; however, not all herbs are suitable to take for long periods of time. Some people take herbs such as senna and *cascara sagrada*, which are incredibly powerful and may be beneficial for acute problems, but they are too aggressive for cleansing the bowels over the long-term or for people whose bodies are more sensitive. I have selected herbs that are also powerful, but lack the harsh action of senna and *cascara sagrada*.

Aloe Vera[25]

Aloe vera juice acts as a natural stimulant to the colon. Aloe vera has been used for over four thousand years for its ability to heal digestive tract ailments such as ulcers, dysentery, and kidney infections. It is full of amino acids, enzymes, chlorophyll, essential oils, vitamins and minerals, and other nutrients that are beneficial.

Aloe vera is known among herbalists as having antibacterial, antiviral, pain-killing, anti-inflammatory, fever-reducing, and cleansing properties. Aloe vera also helps dilate capillaries and enhances normal cell growth, making it helpful to prevent and heal stroke and other brain diseases.

Drink a quarter cup of aloe vera juice, twice a day. Note that aloe vera juice is not the same as the gel, which tends to be more concentrated. Avoid using "aloes" or "aloe latex" since aloe's strong purgative action can be too harsh on the intestinal tract and result in severe cramping or diarrhea. Avoid taking aloe vera juice during pregnancy and lactation.

Slippery Elm Bark[26]

Slippery elm bark soothes the lining of the intestines and helps minimize gas and bloating. For centuries slippery elm bark has been used as an expectorant and emollient. It is also high in mucilage, thereby offering the digestive tract a protective coating to help heal inflamed mucous membranes. It is helpful for healing disorders such as ulcers, gastritis, peptic ulcers, enteritis, colitis, diarrhea, and food poisoning. Make a decoction of slippery elm bark using two teaspoons of the dried herb per cup of water. Drink one cup, three times daily. Alternatively, take one teaspoon of the tincture, three times daily. If you are prone to allergies, be cautious while using slippery elm bark.

Marshmallow Root[27]

Marshmallow root soothes the mucous membranes of the digestive tract, and acts as a natural anti-inflammatory. It helps to gently eliminate waste material from the intestines. Boil one teaspoon of dried marshmallow root per cup of water for ten to fifteen minutes. Drink one cup, three times daily.

Rhubarb Root[28]

Long used by the Chinese, rhubarb root has numerous medicinal properties. This root alleviates diarrhea, and reduces stomach and intestinal discomfort. It also helps loosen old fecal matter from the intestines. Boil a half-teaspoon of dried root per cup of water for ten minutes. Take one tablespoon at a time, and up to one cup daily. Alternatively, take one-quarter teaspoon of tincture daily.

HERBS FOR CLEANSING YOUR LIVER

As you learned earlier, the liver maintains the massive responsibility of neutralizing toxins and assisting the bowels with their elimination before the toxins can cross the blood-brain barrier. So it is important to keep your liver in tip-top shape.

There are many powerful herbs that help the liver improve its capacity to handle the body's toxic load. Some of the best ones include milk thistle, dandelion root, globe artichoke, turmeric, slippery elm, greater celandine, balmony, barberry, black root, blue flag, boldo, fringetree bark, vervain, and wahoo. If you are pregnant or have a serious health condition, please consult a medical doctor before using any herbs. Consult an herbalist before combining two or more herbs or while on medication. Avoid long-term use of any herb (longer than three weeks) without first consulting a qualified herbalist.

Milk Thistle (*Silybum marianum*)

The primary medicinal ingredient in milk thistle is called "silymarin." This compound protects the liver by inhibiting substances in the liver that cause liver cell damage. Silymarin also stimulates liver cell regeneration to help the liver rebuild if it has been damaged by toxins.[29]

Silymarin also helps to prevent the depletion of glutathione—one of the most critical nutrients for liver detoxification and one that is commonly deficient in people suffering from brain disorders. Alcohol and many synthetic chemicals deplete glutathione in the body.

With more than one hundred studies that successfully demonstrate milk thistle's liver protecting and regenerating properties,[30] milk thistle makes an excellent choice for cleansing and rebuilding the liver. Milk thistle has proven itself helpful for easing symptoms of hepatitis, cirrhosis, liver damage, cholestasis (bile stagnation), and alcohol- and chemical-induced fatty liver. Silymarin also stimulates hepatocytes (liver cells) to replace diseased tissue. A one-month study involving 129 patients showed that milk thistle brought a fifty percent improvement in the symptoms of toxic-metabolic liver damage, fatty degeneration of the liver, liver enlargement, and chronic hepatitis.[31]

Another ingredient in milk thistle, silybin, is believed to protect the genetic material within the liver cells, thereby improving the synthesis of proteins in the liver and reducing the risk of liver cancer.[32] Milk thistle helps soothe the mucous membranes, which is helpful if gallstones or inflammation of the gallbladder are present. Milk thistle increases liver enzyme production, repairs damaged liver tissue, and blocks the damaging effects of some toxins.

In one study, silymarin extracted from milk thistle protected the livers of animals that were given large doses of the common painkiller, acetaminophen, from damage. In another study, silymarin minimized the damage from long-term exposure to several toxic industrial chemicals, including toluene (commonly found in nail polish) and xylene. Initially, workers had abnormal levels of liver enzymes, indicating damage. After taking 140 milligrams of silymarin, three times per day, their liver enzymes normalized.

Silymarin in milk thistle seeds is not very water-soluble so does not extract well into tea. Instead, take a standardized extract containing about 140 milligrams of silymarin for liver cleansing and protection.

Dandelion Root (*Taraxacum officinale*)

Nature grows a liver cleansing pharmacy every spring. It is the dreaded weed that most people curse as it pokes its yellow-flowered head through the green of their lawns. Dandelion is one of Mother Nature's finest liver herbs.

Dandelion helps to clear obstructions and stimulate the liver to eliminate toxins. It also helps stimulate bile flow from the liver, which is important to release toxins and prevent clogging of the liver. The *Australian Journal of Medical Herbalism* cited two studies that showed the liver regenerative properties of dandelion in cases of jaundice, liver swelling, hepatitis, and indigestion.[33] Dandelion is also helpful as a laxative and anti-inflammatory herb.

According to Ann Louise Gittleman, MS, CNS, author of *The Fat Flush Plan*, dandelion root aids the liver and fat metabolism in two ways: it stimulates the liver to produce more bile to send to the gallbladder, and at the same time causes the gallbladder to contract and release its stored bile, assisting with fat metabolism.[34]

If you choose to incorporate dandelion root into your liver cleansing efforts, take five hundred to two thousand milligrams daily in capsules. Alternatively, you can make a decoction by using two teaspoons of powdered dandelion root per cup of water. Bring to a boil and simmer for fifteen minutes. Drink one cup, three times daily. A third option is to take one teaspoon of the tincture, three times daily.

Globe Artichoke (*Cynara scolymus*)

Globe artichoke contains compounds called caffeylquinic acids which have demonstrated powerful liver regenerating effects similar to milk thistle.[35] Substantial research shows caffeylquinic acids' capacity to protect and regenerate the liver and eliminate toxins from the blood. It has been helpful in cases of liver insufficiency, liver damage, liver diseases, poor digestion, gallstones, and chronic constipation. This compound has also helped lower cholesterol and triglycerides. Globe artichoke is usually found in capsule form. Doses range from three hundred to five hundred milligrams daily.

Turmeric

In addition to it anti-inflammatory effects for the brain directly, turmeric helps regenerate liver cells and cleanse it of toxins before they find their way to the brain. Turmeric also increases the production of bile to help expel toxins and may help reduce liver inflammation. Turmeric has also been shown to increase levels of two liver-supporting enzymes that promote liver detoxification reactions, all the while decreasing cholesterol, and pain and inflammation in the body. There are numerous ways to benefit from the healing properties of turmeric. You learned about a turmeric-honey water mixture earlier, and that turmeric also comes in capsules and tablets, sometimes under the label, "curcumin," which is the key ingredient in turmeric. You can follow the Indian lead and cook with turmeric to create some delicious curry dishes. James Duke, PhD, one of the world's foremost herbal experts, recommends the following tea combination for the liver in his book, *The Green Pharmacy*. Mix to taste: licorice, dandelion, chicory, turmeric, and ginger. Store in a jar and use one teaspoonful of herb per cup of boiling water to make a tea. Drink one cup, three times daily.

Slippery Elm

Slippery elm bark is good for problems with the mucous membranes of the digestive tract. People with severely toxic livers and abnormal bile production sometimes suffer from irritations of the mucous membranes. Make a decoction of slippery elm bark using two teaspoons of dried herb per cup of water. Drink one cup, three times daily. Alternatively, take one teaspoon of the tincture, three times daily. If you are prone to allergies, be cautious while using slippery elm bark.

Greater Celandine (*Chelidonium majus*)

All parts of this plant, roots, stems, leaves, and flowers, offer medicinal properties that are helpful for cleansing the liver, intestinal tract and blood, while reducing pain. Take ¼ teaspoon of the tincture three times per day to benefit from greater celandine's liver cleansing properties.

Barberry (*Berberis vulgaris*)

The bark, roots, stems, and berries offer cleansing properties that help with detoxifying the liver and gallbladder. This plant stimulates the flow of bile and digestive juices, stimulates bowel action, and lessens inflammation. Barberry is also helpful for mild to severe liver problems, even those severe enough to cause jaundice. Barberry is effective against micro-organisms, including malaria and the fungus, candida albicans. Use one teaspoonful of the dried root per cup of boiling water. Drink one cup three times per day. Alternatively, take ¼ to ½ teaspoon of the tincture two to three times per day.

Black Root (*Leptandra virginica*)

The Seneca natives shared their knowledge of black root to help Europeans who came to North America. Black root stimulates bile flow and strongly encourages bowel elimination. It works well with barberry and dandelion for liver congestion. Avoid using the fresh root since it can cause vomiting and purging of the bowels. Use black root with care. Use one teaspoon of the dried root per cup of water under the guidance of a skilled health professional. Simmer for ten minutes. Drink one cup three times per day. Alternatively, use ¼ to ½ teaspoon of the tincture three times per day.

Fringetree Bark (*Chionanthus virginicus*)

This powerful liver and gallbladder-cleansing herb is useful even in severe circumstances. It is also helpful for gallstones and normalizes bowel movements. It stimulates bile flow, tones the liver, cleanses blood, and stimulates bowel elimination.

Vervain (*Verbena officinalis*)

Vervain tones the liver and helps to stimulate normal functioning of both the liver and gallbladder. It is not a primary liver or gallbladder herb but still works well, especially in conjunction with other herbs. I have included it because it also calms the nervous system and helps with depression. Use between one and three teaspoons of dried herb per cup of water to make an infusion. Drink one cup, three times per day. Alternatively, take ½ to 1 teaspoon of the tincture three times per day.

Wahoo (*Euonymus atropurpureus*)

The bark of this herb is far more useful than its odd name might suggest. It cleanses and stimulates the liver, primarily by stimulating bile flow. In fact, wahoo is one of the best liver cleansing herbs, alongside milk thistle and dandelion. It is good for treating virtually any type of liver and gallbladder problem, including jaundice, gallstones, gallbladder inflammation, and pain. Wahoo also cleanses the blood, urinary tract, and intestines. In the latter case, it does so through its laxative effect. Wahoo is also good if you feel sluggish. Make a decoction using ½ to one teaspoon of dried herb per cup of water. Drink one cup of this strained mixture three times per day. Alternatively, you can take ½ to one teaspoon of the tincture three times per day.

Yarrow

Yarrow is also a good liver cleanser. Two animal studies proved its ability to protect the liver from toxic chemical damage. Use one teaspoon of the dried herb (any combination of leaves, flowers, or stems) per cup of boiling water. Drink one cup three times per day.

Astragalus

Astragalus is an excellent liver protector. In his book, *The New Healing Herbs*, Michael Castleman cites a study conducted in China, in which mice were given stilbenemide, a cancer chemotherapy drug that causes liver damage. Some mice were given astragalus as well. Others received only stilbenemide. The ones that received only the drug developed serious liver damage, while those that also took astragalus did not. Astragalus is primarily available as a tincture, or in capsule or tablet form. Since potency can vary greatly with this herb, it is best to follow the package directions for the optimum dose.[36]

Herbs are the original medicine and the source of over seventy percent of pharmaceutical drugs before they are synthesized and patented. They hold great promise in the prevention and treatment of brain diseases.

PART

The Ultimate Brain
Health Program

chapter
8

The Brain Wash **Plan**

"The secret of getting ahead is getting started."
~ Mark Twain

■ ■ ■ ■ ■ ■ ■

In chapter 8, "*The Brain Wash* Plan," you will learn

- five steps to build a better brain;
- how to put together everything you've learned in *The Brain Wash* so far and start benefiting from the latest research immediately;
- how to make simple dietary and lifestyle changes that will have profound effects on your brain health; and
- what to do if you have been diagnosed with and/or are suffering with a brain disease.

■ ■ ■ ■ ■ ■ ■

Your brain is a miraculous conductor of the billions of tasks comprising its orchestra. We can barely comprehend just how incredible that is. Why shortchange your brain's immense potential by feeding it junk food or not exercising your mental skills?

While it may sometimes feel overwhelming when you consider the number and severity of the environmental and food toxins you are exposed to, you have an immensely powerful ally in the prevention of brain disease: Mother Nature and her rainbow assortment of delicious produce, legumes, grains, nuts, seeds, fish, and herbs. While it may be tempting to believe what the multi-billion-dollar pharmaceutical industry ads tell you, Mother Nature's foods and natural medicines are more powerful than any drug in the prevention of brain diseases.

It is important to eat in a way that ensures your brain has all the nutrients it requires to be healthy for life. You learned in earlier chapters that it is not possible to have a healthy brain and eat the Standard American Diet (SAD) full of processed, nutrient-deprived food that is laden with neurotoxic chemicals. That type of diet only ensures an increase in free radical activity and inflammation in your body and brain, thereby accelerating aging and many brain diseases.

The good news is that following a brain-healthy lifestyle does not require a huge amount of effort, nor does it require portion measurements, avoiding all your favourite foods, or leading an ascetic life. On the contrary, following *The Brain Wash* Plan, you'll eat satisfying amounts of delicious foods. This chapter will help you to put together everything you've learned in the previous chapters of this book.

Whether you are trying to strengthen your brain, prevent a brain disease, or already suffering from one, you will benefit from the five-step plan outlined below. *The Brain Wash* Plan is designed to be simple and fit with any lifestyle. If you are suffering with a brain disorder, you'll also want to refer to the recommendations for your specific health concern, outlined in the next chapter.

FIVE STEPS TO BUILD A BETTER BRAIN

1. Lessen your exposure to neurotoxins in your food, water, air, household, and personal care products. You learned about these products in chapters 2, 3, and 4, and this chapter will give you some great and creative ideas for easy ways to substitute healthier environmental options. We're not going for perfection here; it shouldn't be stressful to lessen your exposure to these foods, pollutants, and consumer products. Making more informed choices and making your brain health a priority in your life will become stress relieving and transformative over time.

2. Follow *The Brain Wash* dietary suggestions. You learned about many of the foods to avoid as well as those to eat in the previous chapters. We'll recapture the essence of that

information throughout this chapter. You'll learn how to cook for a healthy brain, how to protect your brain at every meal without sacrificing taste, and start to learn brain-building new eating habits. Remember that changing your habits can take time. Some research indicates that it can take up to twenty-one days of consistently making new choices for something to become a habit. Be patient and persistent. It's not what you do in the first day after you read this book that will determine your brain health, but what you do daily for the rest of your life. Even small changes each week add up to large ones over your lifetime.

3. Add plenty of brain-boosting foods to your diet. You learned about many of the best brain-boosting foods in chapter 6. We'll revisit them briefly in this chapter so you'll have a better understanding of how to incorporate more of these foods into your diet. Adding a handful of brain-boosting foods to every meal is a simple and easy step toward brain health.

4. Add specific nutrient, herbal, and food supplements to your diet. These will target inflammation and support the brain's healthy functioning for maximum brain health. It can be difficult to get all the brain-boosting nutrients in your food every day, without missing a single nutrient, so adding in some of the best ones, which you learned about in chapters 6 and 7, is helpful in preventing brain disease and lessening the damage from environmental and food toxins you are exposed to. These nutrients, herbs, and food supplements are like insurance for your brain.

5. Adopt a brain-building lifestyle. You'll be amazed how easy it is to incorporate natural brain boosters into your day-to-day life. You'll not only be building a stronger brain and memory, you'll feel less stressed, more relaxed, and more energetic too.

STEP 1: LESSEN YOUR EXPOSURE TO NEUROTOXINS

After learning about the insidious nature of neurotoxins in your food, water, household, and personal care products, you may feel like it is an impossible mission to lessen your exposure. It is important to make healthier choices, while understanding that it isn't possible to entirely escape exposure to toxins.

On the flip side, knowing the prevalence of toxins in your food, air, water, household, and personal care products is not simply an excuse for procrastination. In other words, saying that "it's impossible to avoid harmful chemicals" and never trying to lessen your exposure is absurd.

That's the equivalent of knowing that your automobile will depreciate as soon as you drive it off the lot and, therefore, choosing to run it into the ground by avoiding all maintenance work like oil changes, tire changes, and filling up fluid levels.

There are countless simple ways to reduce your exposure to neurotoxins and heavy metals that will immediately help you to feel more vibrant, healthy, and energized.

1. Avoid using pesticides, insecticides, fungicides, and herbicides on your lawn and indoor or outdoor plants. Instead, learn about organic gardening techniques.
2. Choose stainless steel or cast iron cookware instead of aluminum or non-stick pots and pans.
3. Purchase an organic mattress, free from fire retardants and other toxic chemicals.
4. When purchasing furniture, avoid purchasing additional stain repellants. Most furniture is already treated. Better yet, opt for organic, natural furniture if possible. As the demand grows so will the availability.
5. Purchase organic produce, grains, nuts, legumes, and oils wherever possible.
6. Spend time in nature and away from traffic pollution.
7. Avoid food containing colours, preservatives, MSG,

artificial sweeteners, or other chemical ingredients and hydrogenated or trans fats.

8. Reduce or eliminate your consumption of the three Ps: packaged, processed, and prepared foods.

9. Purify your water to lessen your exposure to chlorine, metals, pesticides, and drug residues, among other things. There are many different filtration systems available. Consult the resources section of this book for more information.

10. Avoid farm-raised salmon, halibut, king mackerel, shark, swordfish, tilefish, and canned or fresh white albacore tuna, which tend to be high in mercury.

11. Reduce your meat consumption.

12. Reduce your dependence on over-the-counter or prescription medications as much as possible. Talk to an alternative health care professional for more information on the powerful medicines available in nature that will help bring health and balance without harmful side affects.

13. Make an informed choice regarding vaccination and respect that this is everyone's individual right.

14. Choose pure personal care products like soap, shampoo, deodorant, conditioners, and cosmetics. Always ask for an ingredient list even if manufacturers claim they are "safe," "natural," "pure," or "organic."

15. Avoid fragrance of all kinds, from perfumes and colognes to cleaning products and candles. If you want something scented or to wear a perfume, choose the purest kind: one hundred percent pure essential oil. Beware of "fragrance oils."

16. Avoid commercial cleaning products especially fabric softeners and dryer sheets.

17. Minimize your consumption of sweets and sugary products made with refined sugar. Choose whole fruit instead.

18. If you have children or plan to have them, opt for breast-feeding wherever possible instead of infant formulas and make sure you are feeding your body well so that it can pass along the great health you enjoy. Use organic baby food as well.

19. Properly dispose of batteries and electronic equipment.
20. Avoid smoking and second-hand smoke.
21. Choose domestic ceramics over imports that may contain lead.
22. Call in professionals experienced in lead removal if your house contains lead paint.
23. Replace pipes in your home that are made of lead or have lead solder or connectors. If you have lead anywhere in your water pipes, avoid using a water softener.
24. Avoid using antacids. Eat smaller, simpler meals and take a digestive enzyme instead.
25. Avoid calcium supplements that contain detectable amounts of lead. Be sure the manufacturer can verify third-party testing.
26. Avoid deodorants that contain aluminum. Purchase natural ones clearly labeled "aluminum-free."
27. Choose natural cleaning products.
28. Use aluminum-free baking powder and baking soda.
29. Choose organic cocoa or dark, organic chocolate. Avoid processed chocolate.
30. Avoid candles with leaded wicks. You'll usually notice a fine metallic thread in the wick if it contains lead. There are many natural beeswax, soy, and vegetable candles that don't contain lead wicks.
31. Avoid imported vinyl mini blinds.
32. Avoid dental amalgams. If you are going to have them removed, choose a dentist who is trained in holistic dentistry and is a member of a holistic dental association. Virtually all dentists claim to have expertise in amalgam removal. But, far fewer have the training to be conscious of your health during the removal process. Before, during, and after the removal process work with a holistic health professional experienced in mercury detoxification.

Even if you take one item per day or per week and start making appropriate lifestyle changes, these small changes will greatly decrease your exposure to toxic chemicals and metals.

STEP 2: FOLLOW *THE BRAIN WASH* DIETARY SUGGESTIONS

With delicious fish, a palette of colourful fruits and vegetables, specific whole grains, rich nuts, and exotic healing spices to select from, you'll eat well and feel an enriched sense of well-being. *The Brain Wash* dietary suggestions help to limit free-radical damage linked to aging and disease in the body, as well as reduce inflammation. There will not be any portions to weigh, calories to count, or carbs to consider. You will simply reduce or eliminate foods that cause free radical damage and inflammation, while you eat more of the foods that counter inflammation and promote healing. It really is that simple.

You'll first need to eliminate foods that cause free-radical damage and inflammation in the body:

1. Foods containing hydrogenated or trans fats, such as margarine, lard, and shortening (even vegetable shortening). Also, be sure to avoid any foods containing these fats, including buns, pie crusts, cakes, cookies, etc. And, my rule of thumb is, "if in doubt, leave it out." If you're not sure about an item and whether it might contain hydrogenated or trans fats, and the label does not indicate it (as is sometimes the case with bakery items), don't risk your brain's health.
2. The three Ps, as I mentioned earlier: processed, packaged, and prepared foods since they typically contain plentiful quantities of neurotoxic food additives, synthetic sweeteners, colours, and trans fats.
3. All fried foods (french fries, onion rings, potato chips, nachos, etc.)
4. Red meat. It contains saturated fats that are linked to

inflammation in the body. So, if you're used to eating red meat every week, try cutting back to once per month. However, if you are suffering from a serious brain disorder or are worried that you might be, I urge you to eliminate red meat. There are lots of delicious and healthy options to explore.

5. Sugars and sugary foods. That includes cola and other soda pop, "juices" that contain sweeteners, cakes, cookies, pastries, breakfast cereals containing sugars, and other sweet temptations. Fruit does not count in this category and can be eaten while following *The Brain Wash* Plan.

6. Grains containing gluten. If you're suffering from a brain disorder, eliminate grains containing gluten, which, for many people, is linked to inflammation in the body. Grains that contain gluten include wheat (and anything made with white flour is actually wheat), whole wheat, rye, kamut, oats, and spelt. That includes any breads, cakes, cookies, crackers, breakfast cereals, or other foods made with these ingredients.

7. Alcohol.

8. Dairy products.

So, what's left, you may be wondering? Lots of delicious, nutritious foods.

The Brain Wash Plan includes

1. Most fish, other than those listed earlier that contain high levels of mercury.

2. Fruit, including pineapple, papaya, mango, lemon, lime, grapefruit, kiwi, grapes, pears, apples, avocado, blueberries, cherries, raspberries, strawberries, dates, prunes, and other dried fruit (make sure it does not contain sulphites).

3. Vegetables, including salad greens, romaine lettuce, Boston lettuce, and other types of lettuce, radicchio, bean sprouts,

alfalfa sprouts, avocado, broccoli, onions, garlic, peppers, cucumbers, carrots, peas, cabbage, sweet potatoes, yams, fennel, bok choy, fiddleheads, tomatoes, dandelion greens, mustard greens, kale, watercress, sea vegetables, turnip, parsnip, collard, and many others.

4. Gluten-free grains like brown rice, quinoa, and wild rice (which is actually a seed, not a grain).

5. Raw, refrigerated, fresh unsalted nuts like Brazil nuts, macadamia nuts, almonds, walnuts, pecans, hazelnuts, etc.

6. Raw, refrigerated, fresh seeds like sesame seeds, pumpkin seeds, flax seeds, and sunflower seeds (not the salted, roasted kind).

7. Legumes including kidney beans, chickpeas (or garbanzo beans), pinto beans, Romano beans, black beans, navy beans, and many others. If you're using canned beans, be sure they are free of EDTA, a common preservative used with beans.

8. Moderate amounts of organic turkey or chicken.

9. Lots of herbs and spices.

10. Tofu, soy milk, almond milk, and rice milk.

11. Herbal teas, green or black tea.

12. Sprouted grain breads (if you're not sensitive to gluten) or gluten-free breads.

Now You're Cooking for Brain Health

It's easy to learn some simple cooking techniques that will make a substantial difference to your brain's health. How you cook is as important as what you cook. It is possible to not only destroy nutritional value of healthy brain-boosting foods while cooking, it is also possible to turn them into foods that have brain-damaging properties.

Of all the cooking styles to avoid, it will come as no surprise to you now that deep-frying tops the list. Deep-frying alters the chemical structure of the oil and renders it inflammatory. Avoid deep-frying anything. Instead, always cook on a low temperature when cooking with oils or other foods containing a high amount of natural oils like nuts and seeds. Remember: if it starts to smoke, throw it out.

Buy a bamboo steamer for your veggies and meats, and play with adding different ingredients for added flavour. For example, add sliced fresh ginger, cilantro, and Kaffir lime to the bottom of your steamer, then pile organic chicken on top. Slice the chicken on top of a beautifully-coloured salad and enjoy. There are countless variations to explore in your cooking. The most important aspect to remember is to avoid over heating oils, and to include as many fresh, living foods as you can.

A great gluten-free alternative to wheat flour for baking is a combination of equal amounts of brown rice flour, ground almonds, and tapioca flour. Mix in advance into a large container so it's ready to use whenever you need it. Use this gluten-free alternative instead of using white or wheat flour in baking. You can make delicious muffins, breads, buns, cakes, and more using this delicious and nutritious gluten-free flour. One of my favourites is to combine one-and-a-half cups of this flour combination, one tablespoon of coconut oil, one teaspoon of organic sugar (in small amounts it's not so bad), one large organic egg, and one tablespoon of aluminum-free baking powder. Mix and spoon into a frying pan with a small amount of coconut oil gently heated over a low to medium temperature. Don't allow the oil to smoke. Cook for a couple of minutes and then flip and cook for another couple of minutes. These small buns make an excellent and healthy alternative to other breads, buns, and even potato chips.

Try substituting almond, soy, or rice milk for dairy products, and coconut milk for cream, in recipes containing cream. Your local health food store has an amazing array of alternate choices you can make for healthier cooking, including whole-grain flour, gourmet prune, nut, and seed butters, and stevia for sweetening. Select organic meat such as turkey and chicken, wild game, or ostrich when you eat meat. You can occasionally have organic beef, bison, or lamb as well. Just keep it to a minimum.

Another health powerhouse comes in the form of fermented foods, which can easily be added to any diet. Sauerkraut, kim chi, tempeh and Japanese pickled ginger all provide your digestive system with a much needed boost, and their tangy flavours are great accompaniments to nearly any dish.

It is also important to eat at regular intervals to provide an ongoing supply of glucose to the brain, without allowing sharp spikes or drops in blood sugar levels. Maintaining a stable blood sugar level will keep you clear-minded, sharp, calm, and emotionally balanced.

STEP 3: ADD PLENTY OF BRAIN-BOOSTING FOODS TO YOUR DIET

Try to get at least five of the following foods per day:

Almonds
Avocados
Blueberries
Celery
Celery Seeds
Cherries
Cocoa (Organic, Unsweetened only)
Flax Seeds and Flax Oil
Ginger
Green or Black Tea
Kidney Beans and Other Beans
Leafy Greens
Olives and Olive Oil
Onions and Garlic
Purple and Red Grapes
Raw Walnuts
Fresh Sage
Tomatoes
Turmeric
Wild Salmon and Other Fatty Coldwater Fish

Some of the best brain-building spices:

Ginger
Oregano
Parsley
Rosemary
Sage
Turmeric

Be sure to use as many fresh, organic spices in your cooking as you can. They taste fabulous and work mini-miracles in your body.

Try to get at least five brain-building foods and three brain-building spices in your daily diet. Keep this list on your fridge and try to get a wide variety in your diet to benefit from the different active ingredients found in each. You can even keep this list in your wallet or purse when you go grocery shopping to be sure to stock up on brain-building foods.

STEP 4: ADD SPECIFIC NUTRIENT, HERBAL, AND FOOD SUPPLEMENTS TO YOUR DIET

While I am a firm believer in food as medicine, it is almost impossible to get all the nutrients your body needs from food alone. This is especially true when our nutritional needs may rise to compensate for the nature and number of toxins our bodies are exposed to. Your body needs support to deal with toxins. Additionally, commercially grown food often lacks the minerals in the soil to ensure sufficient mineral levels in food. The time it takes to transport food causes vitamin content to lessen as well.

So, it is important to select nutritional supplements that target inflammation and support the brain's healthy functioning. Personally, my favourites tend to be food-based supplements, such as food extracts or chlorella. However, every person is unique and has specific nutritional needs that may differ from another person. So, you may need to reread the information presented on nutritional and food supplements, and herbs to help you determine the best ones for you. Ideally, work with a qualified holistic doctor or clinical nutritionist to help you.

As you learned in chapter 6, my top five supplement picks for just about everyone are alpha lipoic acid, CoQ10, chlorella, Cellfood, and probiotics. In addition, most people would benefit from taking a multivitamin and mineral, B-complex vitamins, and blueberry, cherry, and grape extract.

However, selecting additional nutrients may also be helpful. Be sure to choose high quality brands that are devoid of colours, sugars, or ingredients that are linked with common food sensitivities.

Also, your nutritional needs change from time to time in your life. For example, if you are experiencing more symptoms of inflammation like pain, you may wish to add or increase ginger and turmeric to your daily regimen. If you are experiencing a bout of depression, add the supplements listed in the next chapter under "Depression." If you are having mercury dental amalgams removed, choose some of the nutritional supplements listed under "*The Brain Wash* Toxic Metal Elimination Program" in chapter 10 for at least six months. If you have a family history of a particular brain disease, you may wish to take some of the supplements listed for that particular disease to help with disease prevention. Keep in mind that the dosages listed for brain disorders in chapter 10 are therapeutic doses for people already suffering from the disease, so you should cut the dosages down. Follow the package instructions for the particular supplement you choose or work with a qualified holistic doctor for assistance.

As you learned in chapter 7, there are many brain-boosting supplements.

TOP BRAIN BOOSTING SUPPLEMENTS:

5-HTP
Alpha Lipoic Acid
B12
B6
B-complex vitamins

Blueberry Extract
Cellfood
Cherry Extract
Chlorella
CoQ10
Folate (B9)
Ginger
Ginkgo Biloba
Grape Extract
L-Carnitine
Magnesium
Multimineral containing Iron, Selenium, and Zinc
N-Acetyl Cysteine
NADH
Niacin (B3)
Pectin
Phosphatidylserine (PS)
Probiotics
Resveratrol
Sage
Turmeric
Vitamin E

It is not necessary (or advisable) to take all of the above supplements, but by knowing of them and understanding their powerful healing properties, you and your holistic doctor can make an informed decision as to those which would best benefit you.

STEP 5: ADOPT A BRAIN-BUILDING LIFESTYLE

Mental exercise is as critical to the brain as life-giving nutrients, water, and oxygen. "Use it or lose it" is an accurate statement of mental function. Mental exercise even helps in the prevention of brain diseases like Alzheimer's. The Alzheimer's Association recommends keeping your brain active by doing puzzles, word games, taking courses, and participating in regular physical exercise (to get your blood pumping and encourage oxygen transportation to your brain).

There are many simple brain-building suggestions that you can incorporate into your daily or weekly life. Pick one or two of the following fun, relaxing, and curiosity-provoking exercises listed below and add them to your lifestyle today.

Why? Why? Why?
As a way to exercise our mind, Kevin Eikenberry, chief potential officer at The Kevin Eikenberry Group and author of the article "Re-Energize Your Brain," encourages us to ask "why?" at least ten times per day. Most people deny their natural childhood curiosity as they age, failing to ask questions, find out how things work, or simply ask "why?" This simple act will open up new learning opportunities and the chance to strengthen your brain's functioning.[1]

Laughter Really Is the Best Medicine
Scientists tell us that laughter is good for our well-being. Research shows that the act of laughing releases hormones called endorphins that help us heal, boost our immune systems, and give us a sense of health. We don't need scientists to tell us that laughter just feels good! It is important to find the humour in life's follies, watch movies that make us laugh, and enjoy companions who have a positive and humorous outlook on life. What can melt the stresses of the day off better than a good belly-aching sort of laugh?

Take a Walk Down Memory Lane
Taking time out now and then to walk down memory lane is good for your mind...and your heart. Pull out an old photo album, exchange stories with loved ones, or just contemplate the great times you've had in life. No matter how hard life can be, there are always good memories. Walking down memory lane is a great way to strengthen your brain's circuitry for past events.

Do Something Out of the Ordinary

If your day typically consists of the same things—going to work, visiting the same place at lunch, making the same foods for dinner, visiting with the same friends—your brain may be strong in some areas but need new and different stimulation to strengthen weak areas. Try something different! Experience new things. Go to a museum or art gallery. Take a different route to work. Try a new type of cuisine. Listen to music you don't normally give a second thought. Brush your teeth using the opposite hand. Take photos, go dancing, learn a new word, write a letter, wake up fifteen minutes earlier just to relax and talk to your spouse. Doing things that are out of the ordinary routine helps strengthen different pathways in your brain.

The Puzzled Mind

Any type of mental exercises can be helpful in strengthening new connections in your brain and in sharpening your mental capacities. Instead of flipping by the crossword section of the newspaper, try filling it out. As with any new activity, it may feel difficult at first, but it gets easier with time and practice. Alternately, try a jigsaw puzzle or the Japanese mental exercises, *sudoku*. Researchers at the University of California in Berkeley suggest that any activity that stimulates a part of the brain that handles planning, memory, and abstract thinking also stimulates the immune system.[2] So the benefits are twofold: a sharper mind and fewer colds.

Practice Focus

I recently heard a conversation of adults proclaiming how brilliant their teenagers are because they handle so many tasks at once, all while listening to their favourite music. Research shows that focus, not multitasking, helps strengthen your mind. A recent Harvard study found that our brains work more slowly when we attempt to multitask.[3] Next time you want to handle several things at once, stop. Try handling one item at a time. Over time, your brain will benefit from the increased focus.

Massage Your Way to Brain Health

Who knew that boosting your brain could feel so good? Now you've got one more reason to stop in for a massage on your way home from work—massage benefits your brain! Researchers at the University of Miami Touch Research Institute have found that massage helps Parkinson's patients to sleep, as well as improves their ability to perform normal day-to-day activities. Research also shows that massage naturally increases levels of dopamine, a neurotransmitter critical for healthy brain function, and one that is often deficient in Parkinson's patients.[4]

Grasp the Sparrow's Tail

Okay, literally grasping a sparrow's tail won't strengthen your brain, but participating in tai chi exercises might. A recent small-scale study indicates that Parkinson's disease sufferers could benefit from tai chi. Lyvonne Carreiro and her colleagues at the University of Florida in Jacksonville found that patients who attended tai chi classes for one hour each week for twelve weeks were less likely than a group of control patients to experience an increase in the severity of their condition and a decrease in motor function. The study also suggested that tai chi significantly reduces a patient's risk of falling, which indicates its ability to enhance motor function.[5] Whether you have Parkinson's disease or just want to build a healthy brain, grasp the sparrow's tail. You'll be learning something new and maybe even becoming more graceful in the process.

Hit the Books

Think you can't teach an old dog new tricks? No matter what your age, heading back to school could be helpful for your brain's health. A study found that highly educated people appear to have a lower risk of developing Alzheimer's disease. Professor Yaakov Stern and colleagues at Columbia University in New York conducted a series of brain imaging experiments on nineteen people with IQs ranging from below to above average. Their results showed that people who are better-educated and more intelligent use their brains differently. Functional magnetic resonance imaging, which monitors brain cell activity, demonstrated that people with higher intelligence displayed more activity in the frontal lobes of the brain.[6]

Numerous earlier studies have shown that people who keep their minds active throughout their lifetimes have a lower risk of Alzheimer's disease. This research led to the theory called "cognitive reserve" that purports that some people have an extra reserve of brain cells and can therefore tolerate more damage. Based on more recent research, however, this theory may not be accurate. The new research suggests that it is not how many brain cells you have, but how you use them that matters.[7]

Playing Is Not Just for Kids

Going outside to play might be a good brain-health habit for adults too. Playing or participating in hobbies not only boosts your spirit but it can help you learn new things and activate different parts of your brain. Not sure what to do? Get a "word-a-day" calendar and learn one new word every day. Take up knitting. Learn a new card game. Learn a foreign language. Take an adult education class in a new subject: singing, guitar lessons, reflexology, or painting. Or try dancing. Because all those steps and turns force your brain to make quick decisions, dancing can strengthen your brain. Researchers at the Albert Einstein Center in New York found that dancing just three to four times a week reduces the risk of dementia by seventy-six percent.[8]

Taking Strides toward Brain Health

Add two more reasons to participate in physical exercise to your growing list. Since exercise gets your blood pumping and your blood carries oxygen, exercise helps bring more oxygen to your brain. Without adequate oxygen supply, your brain would starve and stop functioning adequately. Even more profound is that research shows that exercise can protect the brain against environmental toxins.

Research by scientists at St. Jude Children's Research Hospital, published in *Molecular Brain Research*, suggests that exercise provides protection against the onset of Parkinson's disease. In the study, researchers showed that sustained exercise for a least three months prevented cell death in the *substantia nigra* in adult mice. Parkinson's disease affects this area of the brain. The mice that underwent long-term exercise showed an increase in production of a naturally-occurring chemical called "glial-derived neurotrophic factor" (GDNF), which helps maintain the health of nerves and the brain against highly reactive free radicals. After three months, the amount of GDNF in the mice in the cages with exercise wheels increased 350 percent over the mice kept in standard cages.

In a *Science Daily* article featuring this important study, Richard J. Smeyne, PhD, associate member in St. Jude Developmental Neurobiology and senior author of the *Molecular Brain Research Report*, states, "If we can extend these findings to humans we could suggest that it's never too late for adults to benefit from the protection exercise offers against damage to the *substantia nigra* caused by environmental toxins."

What's more, it is reasonable to extend exercise's protective effects against environmental toxins to other free-radical-related diseases such as stroke, seizures, and other brain disorders linked to free radical damage.

But, you don't have to run on an exercise wheel. There are many exercise options that offer the same protective effects. Don't like exercising at the local gym? Find something active that you find fun. Go for a walk by the river or in a park. Try skipping outside. Join a yoga, tai chi, or qigong class. This will help improve your brain's functioning twofold: the extra oxygen will nourish your brain cells, and learning a new activity will stimulate dormant brain cells to start working.

Let a Little Sun Shine In

In a study reported in the *British Medical Journal*, researchers found that children and adolescents who had high sun exposure had a decreased risk of multiple sclerosis (MS) later in life. Researchers concluded that insufficient exposure to ultraviolet radiation or vitamin D may increase the risk of multiple sclerosis. Other studies indicated that ultraviolet radiation may be beneficial in preventing multiple sclerosis. The study showed that sun exposure during childhood and early adolescence seemed to be most effective against MS, and that higher sun exposure during winter months, when minimum UV radiation and vitamin D exposures occur, was particularly important in reducing the risk of MS.[9]

Dr. Mercola adds that "it is widely known that the risk of MS increases the farther away one goes from the equator. Scientists believe the mechanism that affects MS is secondary to decreased ultraviolet radiation. Ultraviolet radiation increases vitamin D levels and may have a protective role."[10]

I agree with Dr. Mercola's bold statement: "To me the take-home message is loud and clear. Sun exposure is not the evil it is made out to be. It is clearly important to get regular sun exposure to have optimum health and to avoid these types of autoimmune diseases. So parents, let your kids out in the sun, just monitor them carefully to make sure they don't get burned. Additionally, sunscreen may not be a good idea. The active ingredient in sunscreen has been linked to cancer and will actually block the beneficial UV rays that produce vitamins and protect against autoimmune diseases."[11]

Sleep Your Way to a Better Brain
Sounds too good to be true, but because your brain requires so much energy to function properly, it also requires adequate sleep. Sleep allows your brain to process and organize the information it acquired during the day.

Volunteering Is Good for Your Brain
Help out in your community. Volunteering, or just offering a helping hand whenever possible, may be helpful for your brain. "Good Samaritans" have been found to have lower stress levels and a sense of well-being, factors that add up to better overall health, including brain health.[12] When we help others, we often find we receive the greatest benefits and may even reduce the likelihood of suffering from depression.

A recent study indicates that people who have been diagnosed with depression are three times more likely to develop Parkinson's disease later in life. Researchers at Maastricht University in the Netherlands revealed that 1.4 percent of people diagnosed with depression between

1975 and 1990 had developed the neurodegenerative disease by 2000, compared with 0.4 percent of the control group.[13] Studies show that Parkinson's patients may have low levels of serotonin before they start to experience the motor symptoms characteristic of the disease. Low serotonin levels are also seen in people suffering from depression, causing researchers to suspect that in some cases depression may actually be an early symptom of Parkinson's disease.[14]

Stress Busting

Stress can cause a significant decline in the energy available for the brain, resulting in memory loss, particularly if the stress is chronic, or if a person has been leading a stressful life for an extended period of time. That is because stress signals the adrenal glands, two triangular-shaped glands that sit atop the kidneys, to release powerful hormones. These hormones reduce the capacity of the brain to utilize glucose. When stress becomes chronic, this ongoing release of hormones actually starves the brain of its fuel and lessens brain energy. One of the most immediate symptoms is memory loss or impaired memory. If the stresses continue for long periods, these stress hormones can even sever important connections between the nerves. Whatever information may have existed at that connection may be lost. So, you can probably understand why stress management is so critical to a healthy brain.

There are many ways to control stress in our lives. Everyone experiences stress to some degree or another, but the way in which you choose to deal with it can determine its effects on your body and brain. The most stressed-out people usually don't realize how poorly they are dealing with (or more aptly, NOT dealing with) stresses. Usually these people think they are completely on top of everything in their lives, juggling a hectic work schedule, partner, children, and their many activities, family members, in-laws, outlaws, social activities…just thinking about their lives and the mental "to-do" lists they create for themselves is exhausting.

We may feel that our society demands nothing less than constant work and active social lives from us, but our bodies and our brains need something more manageable. Dare I say we may even need to "slow down?" Sometimes that's just what is necessary to manage stress better—create fewer time commitments. Alternatively, make a commitment to you, your relaxation, and your brain health.

One of the easiest and cheapest options is to simply take time out to do nothing: no work, no socializing, no television (as brainless as television often is, you still need a break from it), to just be. You may be scoffing, "But I can't. I'm just too busy." If that, or something similar, was your response, you are probably one of the people most in need of slowing down a bit.

It's too easy to get caught up in the stresses in life and put ourselves and our health needs last, but it is important to start considering the long-term effects of doing so. Make your brain health a priority today and every day by making some simple changes in your life. I encourage you to read the "Emotional Detox Strategies" chapter of my earlier book, *The 4-Week Ultimate Body Detox Plan*, for practical suggestions on how to lessen stress in your life.

Om Sweet Om

Meditation is also quite effective for lessening stress and the resulting stress hormones that have a negative impact on your brain. Many people associate meditation with religion, but it is a simple technique that transcends religious beliefs. It is simply a mental vacation from the daily stresses in life, whereby you centre your mind and create a sense of peacefulness. The rewards are incredible.

In a study of forty-eight employees at a biotechnology company, half were trained in meditation and practised it for one hour a day, six days a week, using guided meditations that had been prerecorded on audiotapes. The other half of the participants did not meditate. Dr. Richard J. Davidson, of the University of Wisconsin, found that the people who meditated had greater electrical activity in their brains than the people who did not meditate. Some of the effects of meditation continued for up to four months after the participants stopped meditating.[15]

Other studies link meditation to improved mood and immune system activity, a decrease in potentially harmful stress hormones, and reversed effects of chronic stress.[16]

Meditation is simple to learn, requires no expensive equipment, and can be done almost anywhere. All that is needed is a commitment and a small amount of time. While participants in the study mentioned above practised for one hour a day, even a few minutes daily will be helpful.

You can choose breathing meditation, walking meditation, sitting meditation, mindfulness meditation, guided meditation, visualization, or prayer. Turn to the resources section of this book for some fabulous meditation guides that will walk you through the techniques. But don't wait for the books—anyone can meditate, right now!

Commit to meditation for at least ten minutes per day. Simply let thoughts that come to your mind go. Don't try to force your thoughts to disappear. Simply acknowledge thoughts and let them go. If your thoughts come back, acknowledge them again. Let them go again. Do this as often as needed. Meditation is like any other activity. Most of us need practice and patience to get the hang of it.

▨ ▨ ▨ ▨ ▨ ▨ ▨

Here is a simple meditation exercise:
You can play peaceful background music while performing this meditation or you can have silence, whichever you prefer.

1. Sit in a comfortable position where you will not be disturbed. If you have children, it is important to teach them to respect your quiet time. Taking time to recharge and release stress will allow you to be a better parent. Close your eyes. Keep your head upright and shoulders relaxed.
2. Begin by breathing deeply and steadily. Do not force your breathing. Simply breathe as deeply as you can comfortably. Observe your breath.
3. Begin to allow your breath to expand your abdomen. Comfortably expand your abdomen with each inhalation

and then release the abdomen with every exhalation.
4. Continue breathing deeply for at least five
   minutes, the longer the better.

Practise this meditation daily, increasing the amount
of time each day. You can also purchase excellent guided meditation CDs, cassettes, videos, and
DVDs to help with your meditation practice.[17]

■ ■ ■ ■ ■ ■ ■

Love Is in the Air

Anyone who has ever been in love knows that love is good for your health. Research also shows that when people feel loved, they live longer, feel happier, have better health, make more money, have better cardiovascular health, and are less prone to depression.[18] No love interest in your life? Start by learning to love yourself.

I believe that experiencing love from another person is the outcome of believing that you are worth the love, attention, and appreciation that another human being will have for you. No one says that learning to love yourself is a straight and easy road. For most people it may be more accurate to describe it as a twisty, turny, mountain road with lots of climbs uphill and quick descents. Next time you're quick to think of your "flaws" or imperfections, stop and attempt to see the positive in your life. In other words, if you hate your nose and you're in the habit of criticizing it every time you look in the mirror, look at something you like about yourself instead…maybe you like your eyes or hair colour. Learning to love your self is worth the effort.

Just Breathe

Start taking a few deep breaths at particular points in the day to remind yourself to breathe deeply more often. You can breathe deeply while waiting at stoplights, bus stops, and at points throughout your workday. Research shows that breathing deeply for even thirty seconds can significantly lower stress hormones circulating in your blood that would otherwise have a potentially negative impact on your brain.

With a conscious effort to add a few brain-building lifestyle suggestions from Step 5 into your daily or weekly routine, you'll reduce stress, improve your ability to relax, feel more energy, and you'll be taking big strides toward brain health.

Following *The Brain Wash* Plan is easier than you might expect. Plus, you'll feel better than ever as your body purges toxins, creates healthy new cells, and repairs damage. *The Brain Wash* Plan gives you a powerful tool to lessen your chances of suffering from a brain disease in your life. If you are already suffering from a brain disorder, it offers you the opportunity to lessen your suffering, reverse damage, and potentially extend your lifespan.

chapter
9

The Brain Wash Plan for Specific Brain Diseases

"The greatest discovery of my generation is that man can alter his life simply by altering his attitude of mind."

~ William James

▪ ▪ ▪ ▪ ▪ ▪ ▪

In chapter 9, "*The Brain Wash* Plan for Specific Brain Diseases," you will learn

- how to use *The Brain Wash* Metal Elimination Program to lessen your body's toxic load from heavy metals;
- about natural foods, nutritional supplements, herbs, homeopathics, and lifestyle considerations for the following brain diseases:

  - Amyotrophic Lateral Sclerosis (ALS);
  - Alzheimer's Disease;
  - Attention Deficit Hyperactivity Disorder;
  - Autism;
  - Chronic Fatigue Syndrome
  - Depression;
  - Multiple Chemical Sensitivity;
  - Multiple Sclerosis;
  - Parkinson's Disease; and
  - Stroke.

▪ ▪ ▪ ▪ ▪ ▪ ▪

Because the brain is such a delicate organ, albeit incredibly powerful in its capacity to handle billions of functions, it is sometimes susceptible to damage that can result in many different types of brain diseases, including Alzheimer's, Parkinson's, amyotrophic lateral sclerosis (also known as Lou Gehrig's disease), stroke, and many others.

But, unlike many medical doctors and neurologists across North America might suggest, there IS something you can do. While genetics plays a part in virtually all illnesses, so does diet, lifestyle, stress, and other factors, all of which can easily be modified.

Changing one's lifestyle or diet may take some effort, but the result is an increased feeling of well-being, and frequently symptom reduction or elimination. For each of the disorders listed below, I will provide specific dietary, supplement, and lifestyle suggestions in chapter 10, but I encourage you to read through the entire book to benefit fully from *The Brain Wash*, rather than just skipping ahead to that chapter. But first, let's take a look at some of the most common brain diseases and what happens with each.

The common mantra of medical doctors consulting with patients suffering from brain diseases is, "There's nothing we can do." Yet, some of the world's leading neurologists and experts in natural medicine have substantial scientific evidence that this hopeless medical message is needless at best and does nothing to preserve the lives, and quality of life, of millions of people. The reality is that natural medicine is providing great promise in brain disease. There is no need to wait as your condition worsens when there are many natural remedies that have few or no side effects.

For disorders mentioned in this chapter, the disease-specific dietary and supplement suggestions can be incorporated into the overall *Brain Wash* Plan. Do not exceed dosage suggestions without first consulting your doctor. If you are taking a supplement as part of the overall *Brain Wash* Plan and the same supplement is suggested for your specific disorders, do not double your dose; instead stick to the dosage suggestions in this chapter. The same is true if you are taking numerous supplements with the same nutrients—be sure not to exceed maximum doses.

Due to the serious nature of these diseases it is important to work with a qualified health care professional to obtain the best assistance possible. It is important to work with a medical doctor who can follow your overall health. However, many medical doctors simply do not have the time or interest to follow the research on natural remedies and wrongly believe them to be ineffective. I've condensed the latest research on the effectiveness of natural foods and supplements for specific brain diseases. Before taking any supplements it is important to check with your doctor or pharmacist to prevent any drug-herb or drug-nutritional supplement interactions.

NATURAL MEDICINE FOR AMYOTROPHIC LATERAL SCLEROSIS (ALS, OR LOU GEHRIG'S DISEASE)

Amyotrophic lateral sclerosis, ALS for short, was first recorded when baseball great Lou Gehrig developed the disease in the 1930s. It is most often diagnosed between the ages of fifty-five and seventy-five, though even teenagers have been identified with this disorder, the incidence of which is increasing at an alarming rate. Currently, there are approximately six thousand cases of ALS in Canada[1] but as the baby boomer population ages, it is predicted that one in four families will have a member with Alzheimer's, Parkinson's, or ALS by 2020.

Symptoms of the disease in its early stages vary but common ones include arm or leg weakness, difficulty with speech or swallowing, stiffness of a limb, wasting or twitching of muscles, and shortness of breath. Death usually results from respiratory failure. Because these symptoms are common in so many other disorders and the diagnosis of ALS so serious, it is imperative that doctors first rule out any other possible disease like Parkinson's disease, post-polio syndrome, stroke, tumour of the base of the brain, spinal cord tumour, spinal cord cyst, multiple sclerosis, vitamin B12 deficiency, spinal stenosis, peripheral neuropathy, myasthenia gravis, muscular dystrophy, inflammatory disease of muscles, or Guillain Barre syndrome.[2]

While medical doctors offer no known cure, they offer an understanding of the primary causative factor for ALS: excessive free radical activity due to problems with cellular energy production in neurons. Abnormalities in liver detoxification are also often found in people with ALS.[3]

The University of British Columbia, Brain Research Centre indicates that ALS is probably triggered by a variety of environmental toxins, which are unidentified at this time.[4]

David Perlmutter, MD, a board-certified neurologist, author of numerous books, and expert on the use of natural medicine for brain disorders, takes aim at medical doctors who offer little hope to patients suffering from ALS when he states, "Direct and powerful techniques for both protecting brain neurons from free radical damage as well as enhancing their energy production are widely described in our most highly regarded medical journals. Why then are patients and families told, 'we're sorry, but nothing can be done'?" He adds, "Potentially life saving approaches using powerful non-prescription antioxidants like vitamin E are ignored as they are 'cheaper,' that is to say, less profitable."[5]

The primary focus in the treatment of ALS, like other brain diseases, is to prevent free radical damage from occurring and lessen the damage already done. In addition, because exposure to agricultural chemicals has been linked to the development of ALS, detoxification plays an important role in the treatment of the disease. It is also essential to make sure that neurons have all the nutrients they need for optimal functioning. Some of the supportive nutrients include coenzyme Q10, phosphatidylserine, acetyl L-carnitine, glutathione, vitamin D, vitamin E, vitamin C, alpha lipoic acid, ginkgo biloba, and creatine.

CoQ10, as discussed earlier, is an important nutrient needed by every cell in the body, including all brain and nervous system cells. CoQ10 provides assistance to the energy centres of each cell, the mitochondria. Research conducted by Dr. Flynt Beal at the Massachusetts General Hospital indicate that CoQ10 is rapidly absorbed into the blood and measurably increases energy production in the mitochondria. In studies of animals with ALS, coenzyme CoQ10 increased life span dramatically.[6] Unlike the drugs used for ALS, CoQ10 is natural and has no side effects, yet is rarely used by medical doctors. Because pharmaceutical giants cannot patent a nutrient, they favour promoting controversial medications with a list of harmful side effects. Two hundred to three hundred milligrams of CoQ10 should be taken daily for those suffering with ALS.

David Perlmutter, MD, recommends using phosphatidylserine (PS) for ALS, although PS has not been tested for use with the disease. PS greatly assists energy production in the cells, including in brain cells, and has a proven track record in the treatment of Alzheimer's disease. As a result, Dr. Perlmutter recommends one hundred milligrams daily for sufferers of ALS.

The nutrient, acetyl-L-carnitine, is potent in its ability to help create energy in brain cells by delivering essential fatty acids to them, and by assisting with the brain cells' elimination of waste products. A therapeutic dose for ALS is four hundred milligrams of acetyl-L-carnitine daily.

Because glutathione is one of the most potent antioxidants, it serves an important role in an ALS protocol. Japanese scientists found a noticeable deficiency of glutathione in the cerebral spinal fluid of people diagnosed with ALS. Because it is well understood that free radical damage plays a role in the development of ALS, a glutathione deficiency could be a causative factor for the disease. More importantly, increasing otherwise deficient levels of this important neuron-protecting nutrient could prove to be revolutionary in the treatment of ALS. Research from Harvard Medical School, published in the journal, *Neurology*, supports the importance of glutathione in potentially slowing the progression of this disease.[7]

Glutathione is also essential to the liver's ability to neutralize toxins in the body, which might explain why the nutrient is depleted in people with ALS. As I mentioned above, many sufferers of this disease have had high exposures to environmental toxins like agricultural chemicals, which may increase the need for glutathione by the liver. In ALS, attempting to restore glutathione levels is therefore doubly important to help detoxify the liver and neutralize free radicals in the brain.

There's only one issue with naturally increasing glutathione levels: nutritional supplementation with glutathione does not appear to raise the levels of it available in the body. Some holistic doctors recommend intravenous injection of this important nutrient to increase levels. Supplementation with vitamin C has proven effective in increasing glutathione in the body when taken along with alpha lipoic acid and protein. Oral supplementation with N-acetyl carnitine (NAC) has also been demonstrated to be effective at increasing glutathione levels in the body.

Supplement with three thousand milligrams of vitamin C daily as a therapeutic dose for ALS. In addition to assisting with glutathione creation in the body, vitamin C is a powerful antioxidant that helps neutralize free radicals in the brain. It is best to divide this dose into three smaller doses of one thousand milligrams each; otherwise, you will likely suffer with diarrhea.

One of the most powerful and important antioxidants for brain disease, vitamin E helps to neutralize free radicals in the brain. Vitamin E is a fat-soluble vitamin, making it especially beneficial to the brain, which is made up of a large percentage of fat. In the brain, vitamin E does some of its finest work, which may explain why it has proven effective in protecting against Alzheimer's, Parkinson's, multiple sclerosis, and ALS alike. In some research, sufferers of ALS showed thirty-one percent lower levels of vitamin E in the brain than people not suffering from the disorder. Researchers at Northwestern University Medical School concluded that vitamin E supplementation delayed the onset and slowed the progression of ALS in mice that had a genetic form of the disease.[8] A therapeutic dose for ALS is 2400 IU. Because this is an extremely high dose, it is best to work under the guidance of a nutritionally-minded doctor, with the approval of your physician.

Vitamin D, best known for its bone-building activity, is also a powerful antioxidant that is important in treating brain diseases like multiple sclerosis, Parkinson's, and ALS. Research shows that a deficiency of vitamin D may have a causative role in the development of ALS and other neurological diseases.[9] Supplementation of four hundred IU daily is valuable, as is getting regular responsible sun exposure, without the interference of sunscreen since it blocks the formation of this nutrient.

Alpha lipoic acid is a unique nutrient in its ability to be absorbed in both watery and fatty environments within the body. Plus, it is a potent antioxidant. That combination means alpha lipoic acid holds huge promise in the treatment of brain diseases like ALS. In addition to being more powerful than vitamin E in its antioxidant activity, it helps preserve and regenerate other antioxidants in the body, such as vitamin E, vitamin C, and perhaps most importantly, glutathione. As if that wasn't enough, alpha lipoic acid also binds to some toxins, like metals, and escorts them out of the body. Take eighty milligrams of this nutrient daily.

NATURAL MEDICINE FOR ALZHEIMER'S DISEASE

Alzheimer's disease is a progressive brain disorder that starts with memory loss and eventually leads to full-blown dementia and death. There are many symptoms associated with this disease, including memory problems, confusion and disorientation, inability to manage basic tasks, hallucinations and delusions, episodes of violence and rage, episodes of childlike behaviour, paranoia, depression, and mood swings.

The Canadian and American healthcare systems are not prepared for the epidemic of Alzheimer's disease that is expected to strike over the next few decades. About 4.5 million Americans have Alzheimer's disease, but that number is expected to rise to fourteen million by 2050.

Obtaining a diagnosis of Alzheimer's is often difficult because so many other disorders have similar symptoms. Alzheimer's affects a part of the brain called the hippocampus, the location of memory and intellect. As part of the disease, neurons in the hippocampus become entangled resulting in plaque formations and the loss of brain cells, particularly those linked with the creation of new memories and the retrieval of old ones. Scientists are still unsure whether the tangles and plaque formations cause Alzheimer's disease or whether they are a side effect. Scientists are also unsure why these abnormal protein fragments, called "plaques" or "amyloid plaques" form in some people and not in others.

In addition, wherever the plaques are formed in the brain, there is accompanying inflammation, making scientists question the role of inflammation in Alzheimer's.

You learned earlier about free radicals and their ability to destroy or damage cells in the brain. Free radical formation plays a role in Alzheimer's disease and needs to be addressed in its treatment.

While scientists continue the research, some topics worth exploring include environmental toxins, heavy metals, homocysteine production, excessively high cortisol levels linked to chronic stress, and nutrient deficiencies.

Environmental toxins and heavy metal exposures are implicated in brain diseases like Alzheimer's. Studies at the University of Calgary have demonstrated that mercury vapours cause a degeneration of brain neurons and also cause lesions similar to those found in people with Alzheimer's disease.[10]

In addition, elevated levels of a hormone called homocysteine are implicated in Alzheimer's. Homocysteine is a by-product of protein digestion and metabolism. Excessively high levels have been linked to diseases or problems we typically associate with aging, including heart disease, wrinkling, and Alzheimer's. Lessening protein consumption may be helpful in reducing homocysteine levels.

Chronically high levels of the stress hormone cortisol are also linked to this disease, making ongoing and continual stress an important issue to address in the treatment of this disease. It is essential that we develop coping mechanisms and employ stress management techniques to help keep cortisol levels more normal. I've incorporated some suggestions to that end in chapter 10.

Specific nutrient deficiencies have also been linked with the progression of Alzheimer's disease. Some of these nutrients include vitamin B1, folic acid, and B12. Low-grade inflammation also appears to be linked with brain diseases like Alzheimer's.

There are several main focal points for assisting with Alzheimer's disease through natural means: First, reduce free radicals; second, lessen inflammation; and, third, detoxify, especially if a person has had exposures to heavy metals like mercury, lead, or aluminum, or other toxins like pesticides, excessive iron or alcohol consumption. These chemicals are harmful on their own but can also promote inflammation and increase the formation of free radicals, so reducing toxins can help with reducing free radicals simultaneously. A critical lifestyle component in assisting to ease the symptoms of Alzheimer's disease is, fourth, a willingness to learn new things; and last, ensuring adequate nutrition to assist the body to form critical neurotransmitters like acetylcholine, serotonin, GABA, dopamine, and norepinephrine.

It is imperative to eat a diet comprising of unprocessed foods, plentiful amounts of fruits and vegetables, nuts, seeds, and fish high in Omega-3s. Organic food is optimal but if it is not available, wash produce thoroughly prior to eating.

Drink plenty of water, but make sure it is purified, since tap water usually contains many environmental contaminants, including some that have been linked to Alzheimer's disease. Opt for a minimum of twelve cups per day.

Be sure to avoid the foods and other sources of heavy metals indicated in chapter 2, particularly anything containing aluminum, since it is linked to Alzheimer's disease. There are additional strategies for eliminating metals from the body at the end of this chapter. Ideally, work with a holistic health practitioner to detoxify heavy metals from the body.

What follows, are some of the best nutritional and herbal supplements for people suffering from Alzheimer's disease.

Take one thousand milligrams of Acetyl-L-carnitine three times per day since it helps with memory and communication between brain cells.

DHA or a fish oil supplement that contains one thousand milligrams of DHA is an excellent supplement to supply essential fatty acids required for healthy brain function and to lessen inflammation.

Take 120 milligrams of ginkgo biloba three times daily of a standardized form with twenty-four percent of the active ingredient, flavone glycosides. In addition to assisting with memory, it is a potent antioxidant and helps improve circulation to the brain.

It is important to take probiotics that include lactobacillus acidophilus, lactobacillus bulgaricus, lactobacillus plantarum, or bifidobacteria, especially bifidobacteria bifidum.

It is also important to supplement with vitamin B12 since a large percentage of the population suffers from a deficiency, particularly aging adults, and deficiency symptoms mimic the symptoms of Alzheimer's disease. A dose of between eight hundred and sixteen hundred micrograms daily in a sublingual form (drops taken under the tongue) is absorbed best.

In one study, fifty-eight percent of people with Alzheimer's disease had significant improvement in memory, and mental and behavioural functioning from taking two hundred micrograms of huperzine A two times a day for eight weeks.[11] Huperzine A is an extract from a specific type of moss. It has been used for many years in Traditional Chinese Medicine in the treatment of swelling and fevers primarily.

Supplementing with phosphatidylserine (PS) improves memory and brain cell communication and has proven benefits for early-stage Alzheimer's disease.

Antioxidants like vitamins A, C, and E, especially the latter, are important to stop excessive free radical damage in the brain. A multivitamin may be adequate for the two former nutrients, but therapeutic doses of vitamin E (up to two thousand IU daily) is important to slow the progression of the disease. Research shows that vitamin E is effective at slowing Alzheimer's disease.[12] However, if you are taking blood thinners, you should not take such a high dose of vitamin E.

In addition to following a natural diet and taking nutritional and herbal supplements proven to help Alzheimer's disease, it is also beneficial to exercise regularly to increase oxygenated blood flowing to the brain. It is helpful to keep an active mind and attempt to learn new things throughout life since research shows that a lack of mental stimulation can be linked to a loss of brain function.

NATURAL MEDICINE FOR ATTENTION DEFICIT AND HYPERACTIVITY DISORDER (ADHD)

Defined as "age-inappropriate impulsiveness, lack of concentration, and sometimes, excess physical activity," attention deficit and hyperactivity disorder is associated with learning difficulties and a lack of social skills.[13] Because there are no laboratory tests that accurately diagnose ADHD, it is frequently incorrectly or over-diagnosed. Many parents even feel they have the medical diagnostic skills to diagnose their child with ADHD. It astounds me how frequently I hear parents talk about their ADHD child only to learn later that the child has never had the diagnosis of a physician. It is important to get a medical diagnosis to rule out any other potentially serious afflictions. Children are not the only ones affected by ADHD, as the disorder can affect many adults as well.

Medical doctors frequently dismiss the importance of diet in children and adults with ADHD; but, a diet containing sugar, food additives, colours, or sensitive substances can trigger the symptoms of ADHD. Typically a strict diet avoiding all synthetic colours, preservatives, and flavour-enhancers is required to lessen or eliminate symptoms that may be linked to ADHD. To people suffering from ADHD, these items are like poison. Even a small amount of these substances can significantly lessen the likelihood of symptom improvement. Some parents wrongly assume that REDUCING the amount of additives their child ingests is adequate to see some improvement in symptoms. However, my experience indicates otherwise. Eating a whole-foods diet, devoid of artificial ingredients, is essential to the proper handling of this disorder, and needs to be maintained for at least a few months to see a noticeable improvement. This diet also needs to be continued to maintain improvements.

Symptoms of ADHD include mood swings, restlessness, impulsiveness, impaired memory, poor coordination, short attention span, inability to sit still, tantrums, difficulty completing age-appropriate tasks, learning disorders, difficulty concentrating, and/or speech disorders.

In addition to a sugar- and food-additive-laden diet and food sensitivities, there are other causative factors for ADHD, including environmental allergies, blood sugar fluctuations, nutritional deficiencies, heavy metal toxicity, emotional stresses, and poor digestion or absorption.

Some of the most common nutritional deficiencies found in ADHD sufferers include essential fatty acids, and B-complex vitamins, especially B6, magnesium, and other minerals. A study of twenty-one youth with ADHD aged four to nineteen found that supplementing with the nutrient phosphatidylserine (PS) helped over ninety percent of cases, especially improving attention and learning capacity. The dose used in the study was between two hundred and three hundred milligrams. PS is normally found in high concentrations in brain cells and helps them to function properly.[14]

Common food sensitivities for people with ADHD include sensitivities to wheat, dairy, corn, chocolate, peanuts, citrus fruits, soy, and most food colours and additives. I've had countless parents tell me that their child doesn't have any food sensitivities because he or she does not suffer from the common symptoms of hay fever, or environmental allergies such as watery and itchy eyes, stuffed nose, and sneezing. It is imperative that parents (and other people for that matter) understand this important fact: food sensitivities can cause a myriad of symptoms, including all of the symptoms of ADHD.

The most common heavy metals implicated in ADHD include aluminium, lead, and mercury. To learn more about heavy metals and their affect on the brain see chapter 2.

The addition of essential fatty acids from fish, nuts, or flaxseeds is important to proper brain function. Children and adults with ADHD are frequently deficient in essential fatty acids. To learn more about which foods provide the proper essential fatty acids turn to chapter 6.

The most important therapy for the treatment of ADHD is nutrition. Many children and adults who have been diagnosed with ADHD may be suffering from food sensitivities and the neurotoxic reactions of food additives in processed, packaged, and prepared foods. I've observed the symptoms of ADHD disappear when a person returns to a natural-foods diet the way Mother Nature intended us to eat.

The following are some of the best nutritional supplements for sufferers of ADHD.

Most sufferers of ADHD are deficient in adequate essential fatty acids like DHA and GLA, both of which are necessary for healthy brain functioning. Take five hundred to one thousand milligrams of DHA and one hundred milligrams of GLA daily. These essential fats are found in black currant oil, borage oil, fish oil, and evening primrose oil.

B-vitamins are required for a healthy nervous system and brain. They assist with relaxation and help to calm nerves, without any sedative effects. Vitamin B6 is especially helpful for children suffering from ADHD, but it should be combined with an additional B-vitamin complex since they work synergistically. Too high a dose of one B vitamin can deplete levels of the others. Children five years or older can take fifty to one hundred milligrams per day of a B-complex vitamins supplement (such supplements usually contain fifty to one hundred milligrams of each of the B-vitamins, with the exception of folate and vitamin B12, which are measured in micrograms, not milligrams). B6 is involved in the production of serotonin, a brain neurotransmitter that has a calming effect.

Calcium and magnesium are required for a healthy nervous system and work synergistically for the best effects. Many people take calcium without taking magnesium, which can throw off a healthy balance in the nervous system. It's best to take both minerals simultaneously. The dose depends on many factors, but typically five hundred milligrams of calcium and 250 milligrams of magnesium twice daily is beneficial to relax the nervous system. Refer to the Resources section for an excellent source of high quality, lead-free calcium supplements.

People suffering from ADHD often have an overgrowth of harmful bacteria and fungi in their intestines. Supplement with a probiotic, preferably containing lactobacillus acidophilus, lactobacillus bulgaricus, lactobacillus plantarum and bifidobacteria, and bifidobacteria bifidum.

Phosphatidylserine (PS) is a naturally occurring substance that is needed in high concentrations in brain cells. It may be deficient in sufferers of ADHD. Supplementing with three hundred to five hundred milligrams daily for a few months may be helpful prior to tapering off to a maintenance dose of one hundred to three hundred milligrams per day.

NATURAL MEDICINE FOR AUTISM

Autism is a lifelong behavioural disorder that starts in childhood. It is estimated to affect between two to five of every one thousand children and is four times more likely to strike boys than girls.[15] Often a child prefers to isolate his- or herself from society, preferring to live in a world of his or her own. Autistic children are severely withdrawn, have trouble with verbal expression, and tend to live in their own fantasy world. According to the Autism Research Institute in San Diego, autistic children also tend to have weakened immune systems, resulting in chronic infections.[16]

While there is no single cause identified by the medical community, there are numerous factors that seem to play a role, including brain defects that may occur during the birth process, toxic metal poisoning, fetal alcohol syndrome, vaccination, poor nutrition, food and/or food additive sensitivities, brain inflammation, and fluctuating blood sugar levels. Viruses and other pathogens have also been suggested as having a causative role, though research is still in its early stages.

Mercury and lead are the two main heavy metals that are believed to be linked to autism. A recent US Food and Drug Administration statement concluded that children are exposed to unsafe levels of mercury through vaccines containing thimerosal, which is fifty times more toxic than plain mercury.[17]

Many autistic children have food sensitivities. Some foods produce inflammatory compounds that reach the brain and produce psychological effects. Often these sensitivities produce delayed reactions, making it difficult for parents to identify the offending food. The primary sensitivities found in autistic children are to dairy, gluten (found in most grains and grain products), sugar, and food additives like colours, flavours, and preservatives. Parents wrongly assume that if their child does not have either anaphylactic shock (like children allergic to peanuts), or sneezing, runny nose, and other respiratory symptoms linked to seasonal allergies, he or she does not suffer from allergies or sensitivities at all. Many of the symptoms of autism are comparable to the symptoms of food sensitivities, although the list of symptoms of food sensitivities is potentially as varied as the individuals suffering from them.

In a study at John Hopkins University, published in *Annals of Neurology*, scientists found immune system responses that consistently promote inflammation activated in people suffering with autism. This led to their belief that brain inflammation plays a role in autism.[18] In this study, scientists examined brain tissue from eleven people with autism, aged five to forty-four, who had passed away from other causes. Compared with the brains of non-autistic individuals, the brains of autistic people contained abnormal immune system proteins, called cytokines and chemokines, both of which are consistent with brain inflammation. The researchers also studied samples of cerebrospinal fluid of the children with autism, all of which contained elevated levels of cytokines. These findings indicate that treating inflammation might reduce the symptoms of autism.

Another neurologist working on the same study, Dr. Andrew Zimmerman, at the Kennedy-Krieger Institute in Baltimore, believes that it is also possible that the inflammation was produced as a result of the brain trying to combat some other unknown process that is damaging to brain cells.

Other research links autism to the disease, encephalitis. Still more research found high levels of nitric oxide in the blood of children with autism. This chemical is involved in the immune response and is documented to affect neuro-developmental processes in the body.[19]

Autistic individuals tend to have multiple nutrient deficiencies including a lack of vitamin B6, magnesium, selenium, and zinc. However, supplementing with these nutrients may be inadequate, since autistic children may suffer from an inability to properly absorb nutrients, which is called "malabsorption syndrome." This often occurs after excessive use of antibiotics since they destroy healthy bacteria in the intestinal tract that are needed for assimilation of nutrients.

Addressing food and environmental sensitivities is imperative in the treatment of autism. Gluten is one of the most common food sensitivities among autistic children and adults. Gluten is the name of a protein found in grains such as wheat, oats, barley, rye, triticale, kamut, amaranth, spelt, and their derivatives. These include malt, grain starches, hydrolyzed vegetable and plant proteins, grain vinegars, soy sauce, grain alcohols, flavourings, textured vegetable protein, and many of the binders and fillers found in common vitamins and medications. Research indicates that almost fifty percent of autistic patients improve on a gluten and casein-free diet.

Casein is the protein in dairy products like milk, cheese, yogurt, and ice cream. Some people wrongly assume that all dairy sensitivities are corrected with a lactase enzyme product or by drinking milk that contains lactase. Wrong. There are numerous different elements of dairy products that can cause sensitivities. Lactase assists with the digestion of a substance found in dairy products, namely the milk sugar, lactose. It does not eliminate sensitivity to lactose, nor does it have any effect on casein sensitivity, which is commonplace.

Because sensitivities can have a delayed effect and may mimic any disease symptom, they can go undetected for many years in people suffering from brain disorders, especially in autism. For autistic patients, it is imperative to ELIMINATE foods to which they are sensitive, not just reduce the intake of these foods. While this type of diet may be inconvenient, it is essential to the improvement of symptoms and is well worth the effort. I strongly encourage parents with autistic children to make this change.

As I often hear, "I totally eliminated these foods from my child's diet" only to learn that the parent actually means, we "treat" ourselves to the food once a week or once a month. By "eliminate" I really do mean "eliminate." For parents attempting a gluten- and casein-free diet for a child, it is important to be clear with well-meaning relatives who wrongly believe that milk is the only source of calcium or that all grains are healthy food for all people.

It is also imperative to eat a whole-foods diet devoid of food additives, preservatives, colours, fillers, and other chemical or chemically altered ingredients. That means no fast food restaurants and no so-called "family restaurants" that use pre-packaged sauces, condiments, burger patties, etc. Once you've adjusted to these dietary changes, the health improvements speak for themselves.

Initially, avoiding these types of foods may cause withdrawal symptoms, as with other types of addictions. This may mean worsening anxiety, temper tantrums, or other autistic symptoms. Over about three months, you'll usually see improvements in symptoms that can continue lifelong. Some people experience symptom-improvement much sooner. Because every person is different, the time required for symptom-improvement varies from one person to another.

Be sure the nutritional supplements you select are devoid of colours, fillers, gluten, casein, synthetic or natural sweeteners, and chemical ingredients. Purchase a high quality supplement from a reputable health practitioner, or use only the highest quality supplements available from a health food store. Because autism commonly affects children and adults, I've included the dosage information for both below.

ADULT DOSAGES

- Vitamin B6: twenty milligrams (in addition to a B-vitamin complex)
- B-complex vitamins: fifty to one hundred milligrams (except folic acid and B-12, which are measured in micrograms)
- Folic acid (vitamin B9): four hundred micrograms
- Magnesium: six hundred milligrams
- Vitamin C: 250 milligrams
- Probiotics supplement containing Lactobacillus (L) bulgaricus, L plantarum, L.acidophilus and bifidobacteria bifidus: three capsules or one teaspoon daily on an empty stomach
- Wild lettuce extract: helps calm nerves without causing drowsiness
- Ginkgo biloba: has a beneficial effect on the nervous system and works well with wild lettuce[20]

CHILDREN'S DOSAGES

- Vitamin B6: one milligram (in addition to a B-complex vitamins) for children age three to six; two milligrams for children seven to eleven; adult dosages for older children

- B-complex vitamins: ten milligrams for children age three to six; twenty milligrams for children age seven to eleven (except folic acid and B-12, which are measured in micrograms)
- Folic acid (vitamin B9): 150 micrograms for children age three to six; three hundred micrograms for children age seven to eleven
- Magnesium: two hundred milligrams for children age three to six; three hundred milligrams for children age seven to eleven
- Vitamin C: 150 milligrams for children age three to six; two hundred milligrams for children age seven to eleven
- Probiotics supplement containing L bulgaricus, L plantarum, L acidophilus and bifidobacteria bifidus: three capsules or one teaspoon daily on an empty stomach
- Wild lettuce extract: helps calm nerves without causing drowsiness
- Ginkgo biloba: has a beneficial effect on the nervous system and works well with wild lettuce.[21]

The following homeopathic remedies can be helpful for some of the symptoms of autism. Choose the one that most closely fits the symptom profile. Take 6c up to four times daily away from food or beverages (including water).

Chamomilla is best for someone "who is irritable, restless, lashes out when approached, repeatedly bangs head on wall, and finds noise upsetting," while silicea is suited for someone "who retreats into a shell, sits on the floor and counts things over and over again, has head sweats at night, and sweaty, smelly feet."[22] Or, use specific homeopathic medicines for heavy metal toxicity, as listed below.

There are many effective natural therapies to help sufferers of autism, including music or dance therapy, cranial sacral therapy, and osteopathy. Some parents have found music and dance therapies helpful for bringing a child out of his or her isolation.[23] Cranial sacral therapy and osteopathy can be helpful if a person may have suffered from a birth trauma or injury that is implicated in the autistic symptoms.

NATURAL MEDICINE FOR CHRONIC FATIGUE SYNDROME (CFS, OR MYALGIC ENCEPHALOMYELITIS)

Like multiple chemical sensitivity, this is a disorder that many medical doctors dismiss without much consideration. They cite "no research" to support its diagnosis or even its existence. Like many diseases of our modern life, CFS is relatively new and was discovered only over the last few decades. But its relative infancy does not mean that is not a real disorder. Physicians need to stop berating or dismissing the sufferers of this serious disorder as having a problem that is "all in their head." There is plenty of research documenting the seriousness and the physiological nature of chronic fatigue syndrome. Physicians would not treat victims of cancer or other serious disorders in the abusive manner that they frequently treat sufferers of CFS.

CFS is a serious disease that leaves many of its victims disabled. Many lose the capacity to handle even the smallest tasks, like walking and minor household chores. Not everyone who is fatigued is suffering from chronic fatigue syndrome. And fatigue is only one of the disease's many symptoms, which include severe weakness, fatigue that is profound and unrelenting and lasts for at least six months, body aches with joint and muscle pain, physical and mental exhaustion from the least exertion, weakened immunity, low grade fevers, swollen lymph glands, weakened memory and concentration, episodes of anxiety and depression, increased need for sleep, headaches, sleep disturbances, loss of appetite, upper respiratory tract infections, sore throat, and intestinal problems.

While it is common for some people experiencing fatigue to label themselves as having "chronic fatigue syndrome," it is important to get a proper diagnosis. One would not label oneself as having cancer without a diagnosis, and CFS is no different. It is imperative to rule out other disorders that have some overlapping symptoms prior to a diagnosis of CFS being made. Some of the disorders that need to be ruled out include hypothyroidism (underactive thyroid gland), anemia, AIDS, and mononucleosis.

There are many possible causative factors for chronic fatigue syndrome, which include viral infection, immune system damage, low blood pressure, nutritional deficiencies, intestinal permeability, impaired detoxification systems, parasites, fungal or bacterial intestinal overgrowth, food allergies, chemical sensitivities, poor adrenal function, sleep disorders, hormonal imbalances, environmental toxin exposure, chronically high stress levels, effects of pharmaceutical drugs or vaccines, and neurological malfunction. The latest research shows that chronic fatigue syndrome, like multiple sclerosis, involves damage to the blood-brain barrier, making the barrier more permeable and more susceptible to toxins and chemicals like aspartame and monosodium glutamate, among others.[24] This permeability could explain why many sufferers of CFS experience severe effects of chemical exposures that may have little or no effect on members of the general population.

There are a number of possible reasons for the increased blood-brain barrier permeability, including having a genetic predisposition, viral or other type of infection, chronic stress, inflammation, toxic damage, and cell phone use. So it is imperative to deal with these potential problems in the holistic management of CFS.

Because sufferers of CFS typically have severely depleted immune systems, it is imperative that they minimize consumption of the three Ps: processed, packaged, and prepared foods, as well as refined sugars, alcohol, and caffeine.

Many sufferers also have food allergies, the main ones being dairy products, wheat, and other grains containing gluten. Avoid these items completely. Magnesium is critical for energy production at the cellular level, and most sufferers of CFS are deficient. Take 250 milligrams two to three times daily.

Most of the B-complex vitamins are required for various aspects of energy production and work best synergistically, so take a fifty milligram supplement of a B-complex vitamins twice daily (not too late in the day however, since they can increase energy dramatically). In addition, take extra vitamin B12, since it is especially important in manufacturing energy. Because of the digestive problems experienced by many people with CFS, they may not be absorbing B12 sufficiently so a sublingual (under the tongue) form is best.

Coenzyme Q10, or CoQ10, is essential in manufacturing energy in the mitochondria of the cells. High doses may be necessary for some time to get the energy centres working properly. Take one hundred milligrams two to thee times daily.

Short for nicotinamide adenine dinucleotide, NADH is the active coenzyme form of vitamin B3 that is vital to energy production in the body. In one study comparing the effects of NADH and a placebo on people with chronic fatigue syndrome, researchers found that those taking NADH reported a thirty-one percent improvement in symptoms like fatigue and overall quality of life, compared with only eight percent of the placebo group. Take ten milligrams on an empty stomach in the morning.

To help counter any possible candida or bacterial overgrowth in the intestines, it is important to supplement with probiotics. Ideally, they should contain L. bulgaricus, L. plantarum, L. acidophilus and bifidobacteria bifidus. Dosages vary from product to product so take the upper end of the dosage on the package on an empty stomach away from meals. Usually, first thing in the morning is easiest.

Siberian ginseng (*eleutherococcus*) is an excellent adaptogen that supports rebalancing of the adrenal glands while improving energy levels. Take six hundred to nine hundred milligrams of a standardized form of this powerful herb daily.

Because essential fatty acids are required for proper nerve and brain function and to help protect the blood-brain barrier, be sure to take three to five grams of fish oil (from a pure source) daily.

To enhance absorption of fatty acids, as well as lessen the incidence of food sensitivities, take a broad-spectrum enzyme with every meal and whenever you take fish oil supplements. The enzyme supplement should contain amylase, lipase, and protease as a minimum but may contain other types of enzymes as well.

Licorice (*glycyrrhiza glabra*) helps increase the level of adrenal hormones while supporting adrenal function. Take one thousand milligrams two to three times daily for three weeks, then stop for one week before continuing this cycle again. Also, if you have elevated blood pressure, be sure to be monitored by a physician while taking this herb.

P-73 oregano oil formula is a potent antiviral supplement. Take two drops of the extra strength formula twice daily, eventually reducing to once daily. Be sure you are supplementing with the probiotics mentioned above since P-73 is so potent it can impact the beneficial bacteria as well. Replenishing the beneficial bacteria with a good supplement is important. Also, be sure that you leave a gap of at least a few hours between supplementing with the probiotics and the P-73 formula.

Because many CFS suffers may be disabled with fatigue, it is important to maintain contact with supportive friends and family who understand the disabling nature of the disease. As part of the stress management component of this disease, CFS sufferers may wish to avoid those who abusively subject them to the "it's all in your head" statement. Reducing stress is important when the adrenal glands that assist with stresses are already depleted.

NATURAL MEDICINE FOR DEPRESSION

While most people would say they feel depressed on occasion, estimates suggest that ten percent of the American population experiences depression severe enough to require medical attention. Sadness is insufficient for a medical diagnosis of clinical depression. Instead, it is diagnosed when psychological and physical symptoms cause a significant change in a person's prior level of functioning and "inappropriate sadness that persists out of proportion with its apparent cause."[25]

Some of the other symptoms that typically accompany depression include fatigue, sleep problems (either insomnia or excessive sleeping), difficulty concentrating, anxiety, diminished libido (sex drive), feelings of apathy, worthlessness, helplessness, irritability or guilt, mood swings, difficulty enjoying life, appetite changes, headaches, digestive problems, and sometimes suicidal thoughts.

There are many different causative factors potentially implicated in depression, including unresolved stress, chronic tension, genetics, chemical or hormonal imbalances, poor diet, alcohol or recreational drug use, other health conditions, chronic illness or pain, hormonal imbalances, neurotransmitter imbalances, food allergies, nutritional deficiencies, heavy metal toxicity, candidiasis (fungal overgrowth in the intestines), pharmaceutical medications, and lack of sunlight. A discussion on depression could consume the pages of a book series and most, if not all of the causes above could affect the brain, so my focus in this book is to alert people to the main environmental and food factors that disrupt healthy brain functioning.

Whenever I work with patients who suffer from depression, I typically find an alarmingly poor diet loaded with sugar, caffeine, colours, prepared, packaged, or processed foods, and all the food additives and trans fats they contain, and poor eating patterns. Poor nutrition plays a substantial role in the development of depression symptoms in most people.

Food allergens or sensitivities can be difficult to pinpoint in people with depression as they are typically many and hidden. The most common ones are wheat, dairy products, and food additives like monosodium glutamate (MSG) or food colours.

Hormonal imbalances are a common causative factor in depression. One reason for hormonal changes is rapid blood sugar fluctuations. If a person is eating refined sugars, alcohol, or caffeine, he or she is most likely suffering from blood sugar imbalances, which can set off a domino effect of other hormonal imbalances. This is a common problem for most people, not just sufferers of depression; however, people are prone to different symptoms as a result, including depression.

Without adequate nutrients, the body cannot manufacture important brain hormones that help us to feel good. Depression is accompanied by an imbalance in serotonin. Without complex carbohydrates from vegetables, legumes, and whole grains, your body simply will not have the fuel it requires to manufacture this important brain chemical. Other nutrients are also critical. Here are some of the main dietary and lifestyle considerations to treat depression naturally.

Because low levels of the neurotransmitter serotonin are linked with depression and other mood regulation disorders, supplementing with the nutrient 5-HTP (5-hydroxytryptophan), which acts as a precursor to serotonin, is helpful to restore healthy levels of serotonin. 5-HTP's effectiveness has been proven in many studies. The standard dose for depression is fifty milligrams three times daily. If symptoms have not improved after two weeks, increase the dosage to one hundred milligrams three times daily. Occasionally nausea is a symptom of taking 5-HTP, but gradually increasing the dose in this manner helps to lessen any possibility of nausea. Enteric-coated capsules or tablets are also helpful to lessen the risk of nausea. You can also take the supplement with food to lessen the chance of nausea.

St. John's wort is particularly effective for depression, particularly for mild to moderate symptoms without the side effects often associated with drugs. One well-publicized study showed St. John's wort as ineffective against severe depression, while dozens of others proved its effectiveness against mild to moderate depression but received little media attention. Incidentally, the former study also indicated that the anti-depression drug, Zoloft, was ineffective but the media paid no attention to that finding. As I mentioned above, St. John's wort is effective for mild to moderate depression. Take a standardized extract of 0.3 percent hypericin, the active ingredient, at a dosage of nine hundred milligrams per day. If you are taking antidepressant medications like Prozac, Zoloft, Paxil, Effexor, or any other drug, you need to be closely monitored by your medical doctor should you wish to use St. John's wort. On its own, there are no cases of St. John's wort causing serotonin syndrome, but because the herb is so effective, combining it with medications may raise serotonin levels higher than they should be.

Ginkgo biloba improves neurotransmitter production in the brain and helps bring oxygen-rich blood to the brain to improve functioning. Take sixty to 120 milligrams of ginkgo two times per day, preferably of a standardized herb containing 24 percent flavone glycosides and six percent terpene lactones, the two main active ingredients in ginkgo.

There are many other factors which can contribute to low levels of the neurotransmitter, serotonin (an underlying factor for depression and other mood regulation disorders), including nutrient deficiencies, drug use (prescription, illicit, alcohol, caffeine, or nicotine), low blood sugar or blood sugar fluctuations, microbial overgrowth or imbalance, and exposure to neurotoxins at home, work, or in the environment or in food.

In addition to the nutritional supplements suggested above, it is imperative to make certain lifestyle changes.

1. Eliminate sugar, caffeine, and foods containing synthetic additives such as colours, preservatives, flavour enhancers, etc.
2. Increase physical activity.
3. Address the possibility of an underactive thyroid, which rarely shows up in standard blood tests even when someone clearly presents with all the related symptoms. Work with a skilled natural health professional to address low thyroid function using dietary changes, supplementation with iodine extracted from kelp, the addition of sea vegetables to the diet, a homeopathic thyroid solution, and other natural remedies.
4. Investigate other factors that may contribute to depression, such as anemia, blood sugar imbalances, candida overgrowth, chromium, zinc and/or magnesium deficiencies, adrenal weakness, or toxic overload.
5. Take chromium and magnesium. Chromium helps the body deal with blood sugar imbalances and magnesium is an essential mineral for optimum brain health.
6. Drink lots of water.
7. Eat organic fruits and vegetables, whole-grains, and lean protein.
8. Avoid refined foods, including sugars and unhealthy fats that interfere with proper brain chemistry.
9. Take supplements. Anemia, hypothyroidism, or nutritional deficiencies can contribute to chemical imbalances that can lead to anxiety and depression.

10. Increase your Omega-3 intake. A study on manic depression found omega-3 fatty acids in conjunction with medication was so powerful and effective that the entire study was halted so that all people suffering from this serious illness could take them.[26]

11. Take a B-complex vitamins supplement. Most of the B-complex vitamins supplement are required for healthy mood balance. Take a fifty milligram B-complex vitamins supplement once or twice daily. If you have difficulty absorbing B-vitamins, you may need to take vitamin B12 in a sublingual form.

12. Supplement with five hundred to one thousand milligrams of a fish oil supplement containing EPA and DHA essential fats. Both essential fats are imperative to healthy brain neurotransmitter functioning.

13. Take SAMe. Short for S-Adenosylmethionine, SAMe is effective at improving the balance of neurotransmitters linked with mood. Take two hundred milligrams of an enteric-coated form twice daily on an empty stomach for two weeks. Stay on this dose if you experience improvement. If there is little or no improvement, increase the dose to four hundred milligrams twice daily. Because the B-vitamins are needed to assist with SAMe metabolism, it is important to take a fifty milligram B-vitamin complex supplement as well. If you are suffering from bipolar disorder, you should only use SAMe with medical supervision.

14. Take a high quality multivitamin and mineral daily to avoid nutrient deficiencies linked to depression.

15. Take rhodiola rosea.

16. Get enough sunlight exposure, particularly if you live in a cold-weather climate or work indoors most of the day. Small amounts of responsible daily sunlight exposure help your body produce vitamin D. Keep in mind that sunscreens stop this natural process.

17. Detoxify the body, since a buildup of toxins often leads to symptoms of depression. See chapters 6, 7, and 8 for more information about foods and herbs to assist with detoxification. Alternatively, I explain how to gently detoxify all the body's detox organs in my book, *The 4-Week Ultimate Body Detox Plan*.

If faithful adherence to the above suggestions for at least three months has not been effective, then you may wish to work with a holistic doctor to increase DHEA levels in your body. Since this hormone has a delicate balance, it is best to supplement with it only under the guidance of a health professional.

NATURAL MEDICINE FOR MULTIPLE CHEMICAL SENSITIVITY

An estimated four percent of Americans suffer with multiple chemical sensitivity. For this four percent, perfumes, carpets, paint, soaps, newspaper inks, and many other everyday items pose a severe threat. Some of the main symptoms include extreme fatigue, memory disorders, and chronic pain.

A controversial disorder, sufferers of multiple chemical sensitivity, or MCS, appear to be winning a lengthy battle against scientists and doctors who've dismissed the disorder as nothing more than a psychological problem. A growing body of evidence on MCS is beginning to show that MCS is a physical impairment with real symptoms, and appears to be linked to the brain and nervous system. As early as 1999, the British Health and Safety Executive commissioned a report on MCS that concluded the disorder is an organic disease and not a mental disorder.

Yet, in Canada and the United States, many medical professionals clearly prefer to dispense anti-depressants when faced with someone suffering from this biological disorder. While some health practitioners dismiss the symptoms as being "all in [the patient's] head," increasing volumes of research identify this disorder as a physiological, not psychological problem.

However, research by organizations like the Environmental Sensitivities Research Institute (ESRI) has slowed medical recognition of this disease. Incidentally, MCS is sometimes called environmental sensitivities or environmental illness. Ironically, ESRI, a "research organization" has board members in pesticide manufacturing and the Cosmetic, Toiletry, and Fragrance Association, as well as other industry representatives who have a clear bias against proving this disorder's reality.

But sound research on MCS is starting to roll in now. Early studies are linking MCS to spinal cord inflammation and excessive nitric oxide synthesis, which is also linked to inflammatory processes. A receptor in the spine called NMDA (N-methyl-D-aspartate) is activated during inflammation. Excessive activation of NMDA causes spinal cord neurons to become more sensitive to substances other than the initial inflammation-triggering substances.

In one study on mice, scientists found that the rodents developed multiple chemical sensitivity after being exposed to some toxic chemicals. The researchers observed excessive NMDA activity and excessive amounts of nitric oxide. Nitric oxide is a gas that acts as a signal transmitter between cells in the body. Nitric oxide can be increased by some pesticides, benzene, and other chemicals. The researchers made the correct assumption that the mice were mentally unstable or hypochondriacs, and researchers were able to isolate at least two possible biochemical contributors to multiple chemical sensitivity. That mice can and do develop MCS is evidence that the disorder is a real, organic disease.[27]

Other research shows that repeated exposure to a chemical or a single high-level chemical exposure can cause nerve cells to trigger symptoms in response to much lower levels of chemical exposure thereafter.[28] In addition, there also appears to be consistent brain abnormalities found on brain scans in studies, with or without control groups, although research has not clearly defined likely causes, other than possible immune system abnormalities.[29] The research shows brain wave abnormalities cannot be influenced by emotions and/or belief systems.

Carbon monoxide poisoning has also been linked to MCS. Elevating carbon monoxide also elevates nitric oxide. Further research may indicate both chemicals' roles in this disorder.[30]

As the research continues, many sufferers of MCS are finding their symptoms are improved or relieved by lessening ongoing chemical exposures, careful detoxification therapies, dietary and lifestyle changes, and bioenergetic medicines.

The best natural medicine approach for multiple chemical sensitivity is multifaceted and includes the following strategies.

1. Lessen ongoing chemical exposures, particularly those that increase nitric oxide in the body, such as pesticides, benzene, carbon monoxide, or other synthetic chemicals. Refer to Step 1 of *The Brain Wash* Plan.

2. Detoxify carefully under the guidance of a holistic doctor skilled in detoxification of toxic chemicals for those with impaired detoxification mechanisms. Ordinary detoxification or fasting that is helpful to many people has the potential of being extremely dangerous to those with impaired liver function, which I believe is implicated in MCS. Incorporate far-infrared sauna therapy into your detoxification program if possible. Unlike other types of saunas, it is not necessary for far-infrared saunas to heat to extremely high temperatures. In many cases of MCS where sweating mechanisms have become impaired, far-infrared sauna therapy is capable of restoring sweating mechanisms' functioning. Sweating is one of the best ways to lessen the toxic load in the body.

3. Make holistic lifestyle and dietary changes to lessen the symptoms of multiple chemical sensitivity over time. Don't despair; while it is important to change one's lifestyle and diet, it doesn't have to be difficult or uncomfortable. It is simply learning how to live more harmoniously with your body.

4. Try various forms of bioenergetic medicine that can be helpful to sufferers of MCS, including therapeutic touch

or Reiki, acupuncture, homeopathic and botanical remedies, energy psychology, and biofeedback. Please note that, while energy psychology is linked to the psychological profession, it is not meant to imply that MCS is a psychological disorder. On the contrary, energy psychology is a powerful therapy that combines acupressure to eliminate energy blockages in the body and their resulting negative effects.

Because there are many commonalities between MCS and chronic fatigue syndrome, you may wish to follow the suggestions listed for CFS as well.

NATURAL MEDICINE FOR MULTIPLE SCLEROSIS

Known by most people as MS, multiple sclerosis is a serious, degenerative disease of the central nervous system. Nerves are delicate structures that have a protective coating known as myelin. In multiple sclerosis, the myelin degenerates, leaving parts of the nerves vulnerable, scarred, or damaged. If that happens, then the effected nerves begin to malfunction.

Currently MS is the most common neurological affliction, affecting over a quarter million people in the United States. MS usually starts between the ages of twenty and forty, but can occur at any stage of life. Two-thirds of MS sufferers are women.

The symptoms of the disease are dependent on which nerves become damaged; however, there are numerous common symptoms of MS, including exhaustion, dizziness, loss of balance, blurry vision, constipation, tremors, staggering gait, bowel and bladder incontinence, numb or weak limbs, impaired speech, facial paralysis, poor coordination, nausea and vomiting, blindness, and paralysis. One common pattern in people suffering from MS is that the disease always occurs in cycles, known as exacerbations and remissions. Some people even go into lifelong remission.

It is still something of a mystery as to why the myelin sheath degenerates in some people, but not in others. Like most brain disorders, the medical community has not isolated a single cause of MS, but there are many theories. The most prominent theory is that MS is an autoimmune disorder in which white blood cells attack the myelin thinking it is a foreign invader. Others believe that MS is the result of a virus or other pathogenic invasion, either bacterial or fungal. Additional causative factors include chronic stress and/or stress hormone imbalances, immunizations, free radical damage, environmental toxins and heavy metal toxicity, poor nutrition, particularly a vitamin D deficiency, and food allergies.

Multiple sclerosis has become increasingly common in Canada and the United States; but, multiple sclerosis is still rare in tropical, eastern, and developing countries. Some research links the frequency of MS to higher geographical latitudes, making Canada, the northern United States, England, Scandinavia, and other northern European countries especially vulnerable to increased incidence. Researchers are uncertain as to why this might be the case; but, some studies link higher sun exposure between the ages of six and fifteen to a reduced risk of MS, and believe that vitamin D from sun exposure helps prevent the disease.

It is also well documented that extreme, chronic stress and poor nutrition can worsen MS, and some experts believe that these factors may also contribute to the disease's onset. Many environmental toxins can create symptoms similar to MS and can even damage the myelin or the body's own genetic material, DNA. In addition food sensitivities appear to play a role in worsening symptoms for those suffering from MS. We often incorrectly assume that food sensitivities manifest as anaphylactic shock (as in the case of a peanut allergy) or in hay-fever-type symptoms. Food sensitivities are more typically implicated in autoimmune disorders and chronic inflammatory conditions in the body.

Because there are many theories regarding causes of multiple sclerosis, there are many natural medicine approaches to treating this difficult disease. The best approach is a multifaceted one that tackles all of the causative factors mentioned above.

The incidence of autoimmune disorders, of which MS may be one, has skyrocketed over the past few decades. I believe this has happened alongside the increased toxicity exposure. It is not surprising that when the body is exposed to toxins, biochemical processes can malfunction. Yet, our bodies are often exposed to toxins with every bite of food and every drink of water. So, detoxification therapy should be a high priority for sufferers of MS wishing to take a natural and holistic approach to healing. But, detoxification for people with such a severe disorder often works best when it is overseen by a licensed health professional with extensive experience in detoxification therapy; otherwise, detoxing can cause more harm than good. For more information, consult my book, *The 4-Week Ultimate Body Detox Plan.*

Immunizations may play a role for a couple of reasons: vaccines contain toxic substances like the heavy metal mercury, used as a preservative, and live pathogens, like viruses, bacteria, or funguses. From a holistic perspective, detoxification and use of anti-viral, anti-bacterial, and anti-fungal herbs may help. They may also help for these types of infections contracted from other sources. One of the best is pure oregano oil, particularly in the P-73 blend. For more information on finding this oil, consult the resources section of this book.

In Chinese medicine, allergy symptoms are also the result of toxic build-up in the body. So, detoxification is important to lessen any possible allergies. In my experience, dairy and wheat allergies often manifest in autoimmune disorders, causing the body to attack healthy nerves or tissues. Eliminate ALL dairy and wheat products. That includes milk, butter, cream, ice cream, cheese (including soy, rice and almond cheeses made with casein), whey powder, and other dairy products. Wheat is commonplace in pasta, buns, breads, baked goods, spice mixtures, coatings on chicken or other meat, and soups, etc.

The herb ashwagandha (*withania somniferum*) helps deal with a stress hormone imbalance resulting from chronic stress. Take between one thousand to three thousand milligrams daily of this potent Ayurvedic (traditional medicine of India) herb.

Because free radical damage may play a role in multiple sclerosis, it is important to eat a low inflammation diet devoid of harmful substances that increase free radicals in the body, which you learned about in the previous chapters.

Poor nutrition, particularly vitamin D and/or essential fatty acid deficiency, is often implicated in MS. Daily, responsible sunlight exposure helps the body manufacture vitamin D and is far superior to supplementation for this vitamin. Sunscreens prevent the necessary sunlight from allowing this biochemical process. Just fifteen minutes of sunlight daily is helpful, even in the winter months.

Research by Dr. Roy Swank, a professor of neurology at the University of Oregon's medical school, has shown that a diet low in saturated fats with the addition of a teaspoon of cod liver oil daily, over long periods of time, can halt the progression of MS.[31] One of Swank's studies was conducted over thirty-four years. His research and its extensive duration offers promise for people suffering from this troubling disease. As early as 1948, Dr. Swank began treating patients with his diet low in saturated fat. Since that time, other naturally-minded physicians have modified his approach by adding flaxseed oil.

Fish oil in high doses, usually between five to twenty grams daily, is best for MS. Be sure the source is pure (devoid of heavy metals), and contains both DHA and EPA essential fats. You may wish to take a digestive enzyme containing lipase alongside fish oil supplementation to assist with digestion and absorption.

In addition to fish oil, take a GLA supplement. GLA stands for gamma linoleic acid, which is usually found in evening primrose and borage oil. GLA is an excellent natural anti-inflammatory remedy.

A full-spectrum digestive enzyme supplement is helpful to lessen food allergy reactions and lessening the likelihood of other autoimmune reactions. Take one to two capsules or tablets of a full-spectrum enzyme formulation, containing lipase, amylase, protease, lactase, and other enzymes, with each meal. Take additional enzymes between meals on an empty stomach to lessen inflammation. When the enzymes, particularly protease, have no food to digest, they help break down the by-products of inflammation, which are made up, in part, of protein. The enzymes also can help the body destroy pathogens, like bacteria, viruses, and fungi, when the enzymes are taken on an empty stomach.

Probiotics, like those mentioned in chapter 5, are imperative to a healthy immune system and digestive tract, and help to lessen inflammation and autoimmune reactions. The probiotics supplement should contain *L. bulgaricus*, *L. plantarum*, *L. acidophilus* and *bifidobacteria bifidum*. Dosages vary from product to product so take the upper end of the dosage on the package on an empty stomach away from meals.

To prevent any other nutritional deficiencies, take a high quality multivitamin and mineral daily with meals.

Vitamin B12 is involved in the formation of healthy myelin to protect the nerves. Take a sublingual form at a dose between four hundred to eight hundred micrograms daily.

Vitamin E is a potent antioxidant and helps to prevent free radical formation in the body. Take four hundred IU of mixed tocopherols daily.

Plant sterols, which are natural plant hormones, are helpful to restore balance to the immune system. Take twenty milligrams three times a day on an empty stomach to help lessen autoimmune reactions.

Ginkgo biloba is a powerful antioxidant that helps protect the nerves from free radical damage. Take between sixty and 120 milligrams twice daily of a product containing twenty-four percent glycosides and six percent terpene lactones for maximum benefit.

Natural Medicine for Parkinson's Disease

Parkinson's disease is another serious degenerative disorder of the brain and nervous system. In this case, voluntary movement becomes impaired or lost, making sufferers prone to speech impairment and difficulty with most movements. There are many symptoms linked to Parkinson's, including tremors, rigid or heavy-feeling limbs, stooped posture, drooling, shuffling gait, difficulty speaking, constipation, and eventually the loss of the ability to perform voluntary movements.

Parkinson's disease currently affects about two percent of the population, but the incidence of this tragic disease is expected to rise exponentially over the next few decades. In Canada, there are approximately one hundred thousand people suffering from Parkinson's disease, with the addition of about five thousand new sufferers each year. It primarily occurs between fifty and sixty-five years of age, yet there are many people diagnosed much younger. Michael J. Fox, the actor, is one example.

Parkinson's is believed to result from the death or loss of function of a group of neurons in a particular region of the brain. These neurons rely on the neurotransmitter, dopamine, to connect this region with another region, resulting in motor impairments. But, what causes the group of brain cells to die or stop functioning? Scientists are still trying to find answers.

There are several proven aggravators or possible causative factors, including exposure to pesticides, insecticides, and herbicides, heavy metal toxicity, brain inflammation, excessive free radicals, poor nutrition, food allergies and/or sensitivities, and carbon monoxide poisoning.

Scientists still don't know what causes the nerve cells to deteriorate, resulting in low dopamine levels in patients with Parkinson's. However, the incidence of Parkinson's in the United States has risen tenfold since the 1970s. This sharp rise may indicate that the disease is severely influenced by environmental factors, since the release of many industrial toxins has also risen drastically over that time period.

In their book, *Prescription for Natural Cures,* Drs. Balch and Stengler state, "It seems likely that a poisoned body system greatly increases the risk of incurring Parkinson's. Bodies can be made toxic from exposure to heavy metals, carbon monoxide, pesticides, insecticides, and drugs; they can also be poisoned by a poor diet or allergic responses to food. Finally, free radicals, which destroy or damage cells are a suspect in any degenerative disease."[32]

An interesting study was published in the *International Journal of Epidemiology*. The study analyzed data concerning pesticide use in California counties and found an increased mortality rate from Parkinson's disease in those counties using agricultural pesticides. The same study found that California's use of about 250 million pounds of pesticides annually accounts for one-quarter of all pesticides used in the United States.

The medical approach to Parkinson's disease typically entails the use of the drug L-dopa in an attempt to replace the brain neurotransmitter, dopamine, since it has been found in diminished quantities in those suffering with the disease. Medical journals and scientific reports are finding that L-dopa may increase the production of free radicals, thereby speeding up the progression of the disease.[33]

Neurologist, David Perlmutter, MD, states that glutathione is substantially reduced in almost all Parkinson's patients. As you learned in chapter 7, glutathione is an important nutrient that helps protect brain tissue from free radical damage. It also helps to recycle other antioxidants like vitamins C and E. Researchers at the Department of Neurology, University of Sassari, Italy, studied the effectiveness of glutathione on patients that had Parkinson's. The researchers administered glutathione via intravenous twice daily for thirty days. The patients were evaluated at one-month intervals for up to six months. Their results were incredible. All patients showed significant improvement and a forty-two percent decline in disability.[34]

Glutathione is also essential to the liver's ability to neutralize toxins in the body, which might explain why the nutrient is depleted in people with Parkinson's. As I mentioned above, many sufferers of this disease have had high exposures to environmental toxins, like heavy metals, which may increase the need for glutathione by the liver. Attempting to restore glutathione levels in patients with Parkinson's disease is, therefore, doubly important to assist with detoxification in the liver and to neutralize free radicals in the brain.

There's only one issue with naturally increasing glutathione levels: nutritional supplementation with glutathione does not appear to raise the levels available in the body. Some holistic doctors recommend intravenous injection of this important nutrient to increase levels, which the above study showed was effective. However, if that option is not available to you, supplementation with vitamin C has proven effective in increasing glutathione in the body when taken along with alpha lipoic acid and protein. Oral supplementation with N-acetyl carnitine (NAC) has also been demonstrated to be effective at increasing glutathione levels in the body.

Supplement with three thousand milligrams of vitamin C daily as a therapeutic dose for Parkinson's disease. In addition to assisting with glutathione creation in the body, vitamin C is a powerful antioxidant that helps neutralize free radicals in the brain. It is best to divide this dose into three smaller doses of one thousand milligrams each; otherwise, you will likely suffer with diarrhea.

Dr. Perlmutter cites his success with glutathione intravenous injections in his practice for close to a decade, and has found "profound improvements with respect to reduction of rigidity, increased mobility, improved ability to speak, less depression, and decreased tremor..."[35]

Dr. Murray also cites studies demonstrating that high intakes of antioxidant nutrients like vitamins A, C, and especially E, may help in the prevention of Parkinson's disease and may offer some therapeutic effects. In a double-blind study, patients with early Parkinson's disease were given three thousand milligrams of vitamin C and 3200 IU of vitamin E every day for seven years, while others received a placebo. All patients eventually needed medication but those taking the vitamin supplements delayed their medication requirements for up to three years.[36] Work with a clinical nutritionist or holistic doctor if you want to take such high doses of these supplements.

NADH is a form of the B-vitamin, niacin. In this case it is niacinamide adenine dinucleotide. NADH is essential in the production of various neurotransmitters and to create energy for the brain; yet, levels often diminish as we age. Supplementation can be helpful in raising the level of dopamine in the brain, making it especially effective in Parkinson's disease.

Ginkgo biloba is a powerful antioxidant that helps protect the nerves from free radical damage. Take between sixty and 120 milligrams twice daily of a product containing twenty-four percent glycosides and six percent terpene lactones for maximum benefit.

Usually, a low-protein diet helps Parkinson's patients taking L-dopa, since a low protein diet enhances the action of the drug. It is beneficial to eliminate major sources of dietary protein throughout the day until the evening meal, which should still be kept relatively low. According to Dr. Murray, this simple step can effectively reduce tremors and other symptoms of Parkinson's disease.

Natural Medicine for Stroke

The most important fuel for the brain is oxygen. Without it, we could not live more than a few minutes. During a stroke, oxygen supply is cut off, causing brain tissues to die, often permanently. This happens because blood that carries oxygen and other nutrients to the brain is blocked or interrupted. Stroke is the third leading cause of death in the United States.[37] The vast majority of strokes are caused by arteriosclerosis—the fatty build-up inside arterial walls, which obstructs blood flow. Heart attacks occur when the artery supplying blood to the heart is cut off, whereas a stroke occurs when the blood is cut off from the brain.

Too many people consider strokes an unfortunate part of aging. Strokes are usually caused, or made more likely, because of lifestyle factors like poor diet, lack of exercise, smoking, and uncontrolled stress. The use of some medications like birth control pills, particularly in women over thirty-five, increases the risk of stroke.

There are numerous symptoms of a stroke, including paralysis or numbness on one side of the face or body, confusion, dizziness, impaired speech, loss of balance, loss of consciousness, blurred vision, and a sudden severe headache.

Sugar and sodium consumption can play a role in arteriosclerosis, and therefore stroke. Excess sugar consumption increases the inflammation in artery walls, making them more susceptible to damage. Sugar is like many miniature scouring pads irritating and damaging arteries from the inside. Sodium increases blood pressure, which can increase the risk of stroke.

In a study published in the *Journal of the American Medical Association*, incremental increases of a serving of fruits or vegetables per day was linked to a decrease in stroke risk of about six percent, making this dietary improvement an important place to start in the prevention of stroke.

The Nurse's Health Study found a significant decrease in the risk of stroke among women who ate fish at least twice a week compared to women who ate fish only once a month.[38] In addition to eating fish, which is low in damaging toxins, you can also supplement with fish oil that contains one thousand milligrams of EPA and five hundred milligrams of DHA daily to help reduce arterial inflammation, while lowering cholesterol and triglyceride levels.

Take a high potency, high quality multivitamin and mineral daily to obtain a variety of antioxidants and important minerals proven to reduce stroke risk and prevent nutritional deficiencies.

Take four hundred IU of mixed tocopherols found in a Vitamin E supplement to help thin blood and prevent cholesterol from oxidizing in the blood vessels.

Ginkgo biloba is a powerful antioxidant that also has blood-thinning properties. Take between sixty and 120 milligrams twice daily of a product containing twenty-four percent glycosides and six percent terpene lactones for maximum benefit.

In some animal studies, coenzyme Q10 (CoQ10) has prevented neurological damage from stroke.[39] It is essential to energy manufacture in all cells including neurons. Take two hundred milligrams daily.

NADH (nicotinamide adenine dinucleotide) has shown an ability to revitalize the metabolism of damaged neurons, making it suitable for inclusion in a natural medicine program for stroke. Take five milligrams twice daily.

Green tea (*camellia sinensis*), in addition to its ability to support important probiotics needed for brain health, is a rich source of antioxidants that lessen free radical damage and promote detoxification. Choose a product that is standardized to eighty to ninety percent polyphenols and thirty-five to fifty-five percent epigallocatechin gallate, both important natural compounds with brain-health promoting qualities. Drinking green tea can be beneficial for stroke sufferers, but supplementing with a standardized extract of green tea's effective compounds will have even greater therapeutic effects.

Research also shows that policosanol reduces total and LDL cholesterol while increasing the good HDL cholesterol levels. Policosanol is a natural compound extracted from sugarcane wax, beeswax, or rice bran wax. Most studies that have shown the highest efficacy from the compound made with sugarcane extract. Studies show policosanol is equally effective as pharmaceutical medications to lower cholesterol levels. However, it is superior to drugs in its ability to raise the good HDL cholesterol. Take ten to twenty milligrams every evening.

Vinpocetine, an extract from the periwinkle plant, shows tremendous promise in stroke rehabilitation. Refer to chapter 8 for more information about this plant. Take five milligrams twice daily as a therapeutic dose.

To reduce homocysteine levels, which are typically high in stroke patients, supplement with folic acid, vitamins B6 and B12, all of which are helpful to reduce this harmful compound. Take eight hundred micrograms of folic acid, one hundred milligrams of vitamin B6, and two hundred micrograms of vitamin B12.

Acetyl-L-carnitine transports fuel into the cell for energy production and helps eliminate cellular waste products, both of which are important to stroke recovery. Take four hundred milligrams daily for stroke recovery.

As you learned earlier, phosphatidylserine (PS) plays an important role in increasing energy production at the cellular level, while improving cell-to-cell communication, making it an important nutrient in the natural treatment of stroke. Take one hundred milligrams daily.

Dr. Perlmutter indicates that hyperbaric oxygen therapy (HBOT) can restore some activity to damaged neurons. He also reports that the former West Germany had recognized the effectiveness of this therapy for many years, and now uses HBOT in stroke rehabilitation so much so that most Germans are eligible to receive a three-week intensive course of hyperbaric oxygen therapy as part of the stroke rehabilitation process. For more information on this therapy, consult Dr. Perlmutter's book: *BrainRecovery.com: Powerful Therapy for Challenging Brain Disorders* listed in the resources section of this book.

THE BRAIN WASH TOXIC METAL ELIMINATION PROGRAM

If you suspect toxic metal exposure, particularly in high amounts, it is important to see a physician immediately. Intervention with a holistic doctor, skilled in the removal of metals using natural means, is recommended. Heavy metals and aluminum can cross the blood-brain barrier and settle into the brain, where they can destroy healthy brain cells and damage healthy functioning. Metals also settle into the connective tissue, which includes ligaments, tendons, and cartilage in the body.

Ideally, if you are dealing with chronic exposures, it is best to consult a doctor who specializes in metal detoxification. As I am sure you must understand from reading chapter 2, toxic exposures to cadmium, aluminum, lead, and mercury is serious and warrants assistance from a health professional skilled in metal detoxification. It is important to understand that heavy metal elimination requires discipline, patience, persistence, and a multi-faceted approach for the best results.

Before undertaking a metal elimination program, it is imperative to ensure that you are having regular bowel movements. Many people think that a single daily bowel movement suggests that they are regular. That is incorrect. You should be having two to three large bowel movements daily. Anything less than two to three bowel movements daily is inadequate while attempting to eliminate heavy metals. Once metals are mobilized from your brain and tissues they need to be immediately eliminated from your bowels, otherwise they may circulate in the blood and reintroduce themselves into the brain, with potentially drastic results. So, it is important to take the process seriously and be disciplined.

Taking harsh laxatives to purge the bowels is not a healthy approach to detoxification. If you are irregular, consult my book, *The 4-Week Ultimate Body Detox Plan*, prior to starting to detoxify heavy metals. If you eat a high fibre diet with adequate water and Omega-3 fatty acids but are still constipated, you should consult a naturally minded health professional who can discuss the possibility of an underactive thyroid gland with you.

Eliminate all processed food and foods containing trans fats from your diet. Eliminate or reduce sugar consumption as much as possible during a metal elimination program.

While I am not typically a fan of higher protein diets, which are overused for dieting purposes, they do have a place in a metal elimination program. Without adequate amino acids found in protein foods, heavy metals can cause extensive damage in the body as they are being stirred up as part of a metal elimination program. Eliminating metals from the body is sort of like picking up a carpet full of dust. At first, you'll stir up some of the dust, which will try to settle on the floor and other items in the room. But with proper vacuuming and air purification, you'll be able to eliminate most of it. Nutrients like amino acids, and many others, act as the equivalent of a vacuum or air purifier in the body. So be sure to eat sufficient protein foods. That includes both animal and vegetarian sources of protein like fish (avoid ones high in mercury), organic chicken or turkey, legumes, bean sprouts, or soy products.

Take one-half teaspoon of a high strength, high quality probiotic supplement, preferably one that includes all of the strains mentioned in chapter 6. Heavy metals present in the body can throw off the delicate bacterial balance in the intestines, which is important to maintain to assist with elimination of the metals.

Supplement your diet with chlorella. Not only does it help balance your body's pH (the scale of acidity to alkalinity) in your blood and tissues, which tend to be on the acidic side in people who've had metal exposures, chlorella also binds to metals like mercury to help escort it out of your body.

As you learned in chapter 7, chlorella helps to remove heavy metals and pesticides from the body while improving digestion and lessening constipation. This natural algae has been proven effective at eliminating metals, like mercury, cadmium, and lead, as well as toxic pesticides like DDT and PCBs.

It will take at least three to six months of taking three grams of chlorella daily for enough of it to build up in the body and start detoxifying heavy metals and other chemical toxins from your body. Remember, studies also show that after the body's toxic burden of the heavy metal mercury is lowered from the intestines, it more readily migrates from other bodily tissues into the intestines, where it binds with chlorella to be removed in the stool. Heavy metals are persistent, and eliminating them takes time, patience, and some effort, but it is worth the result. It is the natural medicine equivalent of running a marathon, not sprinting.

Because of chlorella's massive nutritional value, it is a supplement worth taking over the long term. It helps to make up for deficiencies in our diet. As part of a heavy metal or chemical toxin cleansing program, it is best to combine chlorella with the other nutritional and food supplements mentioned above.

Supplement with cilantro—that's the capsules not just adding fresh cilantro to your cooking, which is not a bad idea, but you'll need higher doses than that during a metal detox. Unfortunately, there is substantial misinformation regarding cilantro's role in a metal detoxification. While cilantro is a powerful and helpful natural remedy and important to metal detoxification, many natural health practitioners wrongly advise patients that taking cilantro alone will eliminate metals like mercury. Most research shows that cilantro helps to MOBILIZE mercury, not ELIMINATE it. Research also shows that without other nutritional supplementation to eliminate metals, mercury and other metals simply deposit themselves in the connective tissue in the body. While cilantro is helpful in pulling mercury out of the brain, you don't want it in your connective tissue either. So, while taking cilantro, always be sure to follow the remaining fundamentals of metal elimination mentioned here.

Have your health practitioner determine if you have insufficient levels of hydrochloric acid, which is a natural stomach acid. Many people immediately assume that they have more than enough if they are prone to indigestion or heartburn. Actually, those symptoms are frequently signs of low hydrochloric acid, contrary to what so-called aluminum-laden antacid manufacturers would have you believe. Some of the symptoms of low stomach acid include bloating, belching, burning, flatulence, diarrhea, constipation, nausea after eating (particularly after taking nutritional supplements), and food allergies. If you are suffering from food sensitivities, you are likely deficient in hydrochloric acid. If you suspect low stomach acid, supplement with betaine hydrochloride taken with the first bite of every meal. Usually one to six capsules of betaine hydrochloride may be needed to ensure that the nutrients in food and supplements are adequately broken down. Always start with one at each meal and gradually add one more capsule over time.

Supplementing with pectin is helpful to eliminate toxic metals from the body since it binds to them in the intestines where they can be removed in bowel movements. Pectin is a specific type of fibre, usually extracted from apples or citrus fruit. As a supplement, it may be found under the name "modified citrus extract." You take it by stirring a teaspoonful or two into a glass of juice, or through capsules. Be sure to drink at least one cup of juice or water to ensure you are getting adequate liquid. Pectin binds to heavy metals in the bloodstream and helps flush them out via the liver, according to Nan Kathryn Fuchs, PhD, a nutrition researcher.[40] According to research from California's Amitabha Medical Center, five grams of pectin daily is enough to flush almost seventy percent of heavy metals out of most people's bodies within months.

Based on additional research, a pectin-rich diet may decrease total cholesterol by twelve percent, and lower the potentially-harmful LDL cholesterol by fifteen percent. Lowering cholesterol by this amount can cut your risk of heart disease and stroke by twenty-five percent. As if that weren't enough reason to take pectin, a recent study found that pectin also attaches itself to cancer cells, thereby preventing up to ninety-five percent of them from developing into full-blown tumors. Studies out of California indicate that taking fourteen grams of pectin daily may help prevent lung, skin, and prostate cancers from spreading. This is a high dose which should be taken in smaller doses throughout the day, preferably away from any vitamins or minerals since it can also bind them and escort them out of the body.

I highly recommend that, if you choose to supplement with pectin, you follow through with the high dose daily for a minimum of three, but preferably six months. Otherwise you may begin to mobilize metals in the body only to have them circulate in the blood and settle into other bodily tissues. After that, continue to eat foods high in pectin to help maintain the results you have. These foods include apples, bananas, beets, cabbage, carrots, citrus fruits, dried peas, and okra.

Many nutrients assist in detoxifying heavy metals or in binding to them to escort them out of the body. Some of the main ones include vitamins A, C, E, B1, B2, B6, and B12, beta carotene, niacin, pantothenic acid, folic acid, biotin, choline, inositol, methionine, calcium, magnesium, potassium, zinc, silicon, manganese, iodine, chromium, and selenium. During a heavy metal detoxification, it is important to supplement with a broad spectrum multivitamin and mineral, preferably one that has been formulated specifically for nutritional chelation. Many detox functions will not work properly without critical vitamins. Minerals are also needed to ensure detox processes function properly. Enzymes that are involved in every bodily function have binding sites that require minerals for them to function. If there are insufficient amounts of important minerals like magnesium, selenium, zinc, or sodium, the body will hold onto heavy metals at these binding sites instead. There is a substantial body of research supporting the use of key nutrients to lessen the toxic load of metals in the body.

HOMEOPATHY FOR DETOXIFYING HEAVY METALS AND OTHER TOXIC SUBSTANCES

Homeopathic remedies can be helpful with any brain disorder, but are especially valuable to help the body to eliminate toxic substances alongside a detox program. For this purpose, I consulted with Tutti Gould, a friend and expert homeopath, who shared some of her favourite remedies for dealing with heavy metals, drug toxicity, and vaccines.

What medical substance becomes more powerful when it ceases to exist in its physical form? According to German physician Dr. Samuel Hahnemann, the same substance that potentially causes an illness in the first place. It sounds strange but this is the basic premise of homeopathy: dilute a substance until none of the original material remains and you are left with its "energetic signature."

Hahnemann was not alone in this belief. Hippocrates, the father of modern medicine, stated many centuries ago that "like cures like," and through years of experimentation, Hahnemann discovered that the most effective way to combat particular illnesses was to deliver highly diluted substances to the body that, in their undiluted form, would create the same symptoms of the illness. The word "homeopathy" is derived from two Greek words: "homos," meaning like, and "pathos," meaning suffering. If this theory sounds too wacky for you, consider this: vaccines are based on the same principle. Unlike homeopathy, a vaccination will deliver toxic chemical additives such as heavy metals along with the substance intended to help the body.

In my experience, homeopathy is most effective when administered by a skilled practitioner. It is a truly holistic healing modality when a homeopath selects remedies for their physical, emotional, mental, and spiritual attributes. To accomplish such a task, a homeopath may ask you many questions to obtain a clear picture of your symptoms and what conditions make them worse or better. Homeopathic remedies are available in different potencies and dosages, which can be confusing. While there is no single homeopathic remedy to tackle detoxification on an energetic (and ultimately) physical level, a visit to a homeopath may be a helpful addition to your program. You may encounter a powerful, healing alternative for specific ailments or issues with which you have been struggling.[41]

Heavy Metal and Homeopathy

Mercury, aluminum, and lead are heavy metals that we are exposed to. The mercury of dental fillings has been proven to leak into the bloodstream affecting the heart, brain, kidneys, and immune system.

Mercurius is used to counteract the effects of cavity fillings such as gum disease, bleeding gums, abscesses, oral ulcers, colitis, or frequent miscarriages.

Sulphur has a broad-spectrum effect on metals, helping the body to detoxify them from deep tissues, lymphatic system, and the liver. Sulphur can be used to clear general heavy metal toxicity as a preliminary clean up. Sulphur is specific for helping with fatigue, skin eruptions, and slow healing.

Drug Detox

Whether drugs are prescribed or recreational, they will have a toxic effect on the body. Homeopathic remedies reduce the side effects of drugs like tranquilizers, Prozac, and marijuana. *Nux vomica* is used as a general antidote for drugs, whether prescription or recreational, especially for overuse of anti-depressants, as it helps the congested liver. A person needing this remedy is highly sensitive to sound, light, smell, and touch. He or she may be angry, impatient, critical, and suffer from burnout.

Vaccinations

Homeopathy has been helping with the side effects of vaccinations for many years, without interfering with their effectiveness. Vaccinations, although beneficial, have also been linked with asthma, autism, and ADD. Thuya is to be given immediately after any immunization, daily for three to four days. Someone suffering from convulsions or other serious symptoms after vaccination should seek immediate medical attention, as well as consult a professional homeopath simultaneously. Homeopathic remedies are usually recommended based on an individual's particular nature, which is the most accurate way to bring about success. However, in some cases the remedies are given based on general conditions discussed above. It is always advisable to seek professional help to accurately determine the correct homeopathic remedy.

Whether you are tackling a specific toxin, or just want
a general detox, you can combine these remedies
with any other detox program, such as a change in
diet, or exercise program, and these changes will
work in harmony for that inner cleansing.[42]

■ ■ ■ ■ ■ ■ ■

*This text was used with permission of Tutti Gould and Michelle Decary.

COPING WITH BRAIN DISEASE

There are many other brain disorders; however, research indicates that
most of these diseases may have some common causative factors, including poor diet; inflammation and excessive free radical damage to
the brain; oxygen insufficiency or damage in the brain; inadequate nutrients for proper brain function, particularly in the power centres of
brain cells; ingestion of harmful neurotoxins through common foods,
especially those called excitotoxins, which actually "excite" brain cells
to death; heavy metal toxicity or general toxicity; and food sensitivities. The University of British Columbia Brain Research Centre cites
its belief that many of the above causative factors are probably common to all brain diseases.

Natural medicine holds tremendous promise in the prevention
and treatment of many brain diseases. The growing body of research
is proving that food, nutritional supplementation, and other natural
medicines are having profound effects on the health of the brain.

chapter
10

Natural Therapies to Boost Your Brain

"The Doctor of the future will give no medicine, but will interest his patients in the care of the human frame, in diet, and in the cause and prevention of disease."

~ Attributed to Thomas Alva Edison

■ ■ ■ ■ ■ ■ ■

In chapter 10, "Natural Therapies to Boost Your Brain," you will learn the best natural therapies for brain disease prevention and treatment:

- Detoxification Therapy;
- Far-Infrared Sauna Therapy;
- Hyperbaric Oxygen Therapy;
- Medical Aromatherapy;
- Nutritional Chelation;
- Acupuncture and Acupressure; and
- Quantum Biofeedback.

■ ■ ■ ■ ■ ■ ■

The realm of natural medicine offers great promise in the prevention and treatment of brain disease by offering natural therapies that help to restore balance holistically: to body, mind, and spirit. The range runs from ancient healing techniques like acupressure and acupuncture, to modern technological advancements such as quantum biofeedback, far-infrared sauna therapy, or hyperbaric oxygen therapy. This chapter is not by any means a complete list of all the possible natural therapies that may benefit brain diseases. I have selected a handful that I believe have the greatest potential in prevention, and ones you may wish to include in your brain health plan.

DETOXIFICATION THERAPY

Regular detoxification is essential to brain health. It can help eliminate toxins we've been exposed to before they can cross the blood-brain barrier to gain access to the brain.

The best approach to detoxification is to determine the organs that may be sluggish, and to work with a natural healthcare provider to move systematically through all of the detox organs with special emphasis on your weak areas. For more information, turn to the resources section at the end of this book. It is vital that you learn how to detoxify your urinary and digestive tracts, lymphatic system, liver, gallbladder, blood, respiratory system, and skin in an order that works best and causes the fewest negative symptoms. A detoxification program should be holistic in its approach, working to balance the emotions and energies as much as the physical body.

There are many approaches to detoxification. Some focus primarily on diet, others use herbs, still others employ detoxification therapies, like saunas or massage. A combination of these approaches typically works best, particularly when the combination is individualized for your specific needs. Detoxification therapy is beneficial to almost everyone, but may be especially needed by people suffering from brain illnesses. If you are suffering from such a disorder, it is important to work with a health practitioner skilled at detoxification therapy, particularly if you are going to conduct a heavy metal detoxification program.

For those who have had significant metal or environmental toxin exposure, embarking on an intensive detoxification program may be beneficial. Consider the New York Rescue Workers Detoxification Project, a program to assist the fire fighters and rescue workers at the tragic September 11, 2001, destruction of the Twin Towers. Using an intensive program designed by L. Ron Hubbard, combining specific diet, nutritional supplementation, exercise, sauna, fluid replacement, and rest, proved effective for over five hundred people who had been exposed to dangerous levels of environmental toxins and metals. The outcome of this study is significant, including substantial symptom reversal, and documented neurological improvement.

FAR-INFRARED SAUNA THERAPY

One valuable way to assist with detoxification of heavy metals and environmental chemicals is through the use of far-infrared sauna therapy.

From the native civilizations across North America to the Scandinavian cultures of Northern Europe, people around the world have recognized the health benefits of increasing one's body temperature. Unfortunately, sweat lodges are not as common as they once were, but modern technology has helped bring the benefits of heat to us in the form of products using far-infrared radiation (FIR). Today, you will find heat lamps, quilts and even hair dryers that deliver therapeutic heat to our bodies. However, my favourite form of far-infrared radiation technology for the purpose of detoxification is the sauna.

Radiation, you say? Yes, I know radiation has negative connotations in modern society and we avoid "all things radioactive" (if we know what they are). What most of us do not realize is that radiation comes in many forms. There is the lethal atomic radiation from a nuclear bomb blast. Ultraviolet radiation, such as the harmful rays from the sun, can burn and damage the skin when they penetrate the ozone layers. But the sun also delivers healing, warm rays, or radiant heat. This is infrared radiation, a form of energy that heats objects directly. In other words, it does not heat the air in between.

A short science lesson helps to explain the heat/radiation/energy relationship. Infrared radiation is measured as light along the electromagnetic spectrum. It falls below ("infra") the red light segment along this spectrum—hence the name infrared. While it is not visible to the human eye, this light penetrates our skin surface and is absorbed by our cells. Visible light simply bounces off our skin. Near-infrared light is absorbed at the skin level and will cause the surface skin temperature to increase moderately. Far-infrared light can penetrate our bodies up to an estimated four centimetres and works energetically at the cellular level. Research has demonstrated that this penetrating radiant heat can increase metabolism and blood circulation in addition to raising our core body temperature. And what do all of these things have in common? You guessed it: they promote detoxification and help to heal the body.

Please do not confuse FIR saunas with the traditional idea of a sauna. You won't be pouring water over hot rocks to create steam and moist heat. These steam saunas can be beneficial but the high temperatures and humidity can create a cardiovascular risk. FIR saunas mimic nature by delivering radiant heat through ceramic infrared heaters. No hot stones, no water, no humidity, but plenty of sweat. The energy delivered from a FIR sauna creates a "sweat volume" that is two to three times greater than a conventional steam sauna. This is also accomplished at a lower (and therefore less risky) temperature. FIR saunas typically operate in the range of 110° to 130° Fahrenheit, while steam saunas can reach 180° to 235° Fahrenheit. Consequently, heart rate and blood pressure concerns are greatly reduced while you sweat out those toxins. The most important thing to remember is to replace that fluid and mineral loss with pure water to prevent dehydration. In addition to your usual eight to ten cups of water daily, add at least two more cups for each sauna session.

If you can find a health practitioner that offers FIR sauna as a therapy, I urge you to consider adding it to the detoxification program. If you can afford to purchase one (about five thousand dollars and up), it is a great lifestyle addition. These units often look like small cabins constructed of various wood species such as cedar or oak. FIR saunas vary in dimensions but can typically accommodate one to six people."[1] I usually recommend people try to find a health clinic that offers a high quality far-infrared sauna therapy so they can try it first before making a commitment to purchase one at such steep prices.

Far-infrared sauna therapy is even being used in the toughest of detoxification situations. Fire fighters at Ground Zero who were exposed to high levels of harsh environmental toxins during 9/11 are taking part in intensive detoxification therapy that includes far-infrared saunas.

HYPERBARIC OXYGEN THERAPY (HBOT)

Hyperbaric Oxygen Therapy (HBOT) involves giving someone oxygen under increased atmospheric pressure. Special chambers are used in some health clinics throughout Europe, Asia, and, more recently, North America. In the former two continents, HBOT has been used for several decades for the treatment of stroke, multiple sclerosis, head injury, and cerebral palsy. David Perlmutter, MD, a board certified neurologist and author of numerous books on brain health, cites HBOT's effectiveness in treating brain diseases, and for the reduction of free radicals. He cites research on HBOT's effectiveness for cerebral palsy, head injury, and Bell's palsy.[2]

Treatment sessions last between sixty to ninety minutes, and are administered in a chamber for one person at a time. Treatments are administered by a trained technician and supervised by a medical doctor. The chamber is slowly pressurized with pure oxygen until the appropriate pressure is attained. Patients must swallow or drink water to clear the pressure in their ears much like they would do if flying in an airplane. Ear tubes can be used for those with difficulty equalizing their ear pressure.

Many patients fall asleep or watch a movie, again much like they would if flying in an airplane. The difference in this case is that in addition to the increased pressure, patients are being exposed to one hundred percent pure oxygen. It can be difficult to find HBOT therapy; but, you might find the effort worthwhile, particularly if you are already experiencing a brain disease.

MEDICAL AROMATHERAPY

Don't be fooled by its natural and beautiful scents; medical aromatherapy is a powerful therapy for healing brain diseases. Medical aromatherapy is the art and science of using essential oils for therapeutic purposes.

Essential oils are the oily liquids distilled from plants, including flowers, seeds, leaves, stems, roots, resin, and bark. Many factors determine the therapeutic quality of essential oils, such as which part was used for oil extraction, geographical region, altitude, climate, soil, growing conditions, harvest method and season, and the distillation process. Many of the essential oils sold by retailers are substandard for therapeutic purposes, particularly in the field of medical aromatherapy, where only the highest-grade oils are used.

Natural scents have a direct pathway to the brain and research shows that some chemical constituents of aromatherapy oils, particularly a class of compounds, known as sesquiterpenes, can cross the blood-brain barrier and increase oxygen flow to the brain.

Researchers at the Universities of Vienna and Berlin found that sesquiterpenes in the essential oils frankincense and sandalwood can increase levels of oxygen in the brain by as much as twenty-eight percent.[3] Such a tremendous increase in oxygen can dramatically affect the activity in the brain, improving emotions, learning, attitude, immune function, hormone balance, and energy levels. In another study published in *Complementary Therapies in Clinical Practice*, the essential oil sandalwood was deemed effective at reducing anxiety.

High levels of sesquiterpenes are also found in other essential oils, including melissa, myrrh, and clove. While still in the early stages, the research suggests that these oils, along with sandalwood and frankincense, have tremendous potential in the prevention and treatment of brain diseases.

There are numerous ways to benefit from essential oils. Aromatherapy diffusers are usually available from qualified aromatherapists and other naturally minded health professionals. The best type of diffuser sprays microscopic amounts of essential oils into the air without heating the oils. To preserve the therapeutic integrity of the oils, it is best that they are diffused without heat, since heat alters their chemical constituents. If you don't have access to a diffuser, you can apply a few drops to the skin, diluted in a teaspoon or two of carrier oil, such as sweet almond, hazelnut, or grape seed as part of an aromatherapy massage. Alternately, you can put a few drops on a handkerchief and inhale the scents at regular intervals throughout the day. Healing never smelled so good.

NUTRITIONAL CHELATION

Chelation is the process of taking substances known to bind to toxins and help eliminate them from the body. There are two main kinds of chelation in natural medicine: intravenous or nutritional. This section will focus on nutritional chelation.

My experience with nutritional chelation, also called oral chelation, spans almost a decade and a half. It involves supplementing your diet with high doses of specific nutrients that bind to toxins in the body to assist with their breakdown and elimination. Chelating (pronounced "key-layting") agents are substances that bind to metals or chemical toxins in the body. In this case nutrients act as chelating agents. These nutrients can include vitamins, minerals, amino acids, phytonutrients, herbs, and enzymes. Nutrients are used to bind to heavy metals in the body, like mercury, lead, cadmium, and aluminium, to help extract them from tissues and organs, and assist with the toxins' elimination. Each nutrient tends to have an innate attraction to different types of metals or toxins, making a combination of nutrients most effective for the elimination of a broad spectrum of toxins in the body.

It is believed that the nutrients bind to metal or toxin ions, which are charged atoms, to carry them out of the body via urine or feces. A beneficial side effect of nutritional chelation is its ability to lower cholesterol and lessen its build-up in the arteries. Another beneficial side effect includes the lessening of free radical activity and resulting damage.

Nutritional chelation is a gentle and gradual approach to eliminating toxins from the body. It is best administered and overseen by a clinical nutritionist or holistic doctor versed in nutritional chelation. A general rule of thumb regarding the timeframe is at least one month of a high-potency nutritional chelation supplement for every decade of life; however, varied toxic exposures may change the duration of the program.

Most nutritional chelation formulas include vitamin A, beta carotene, vitamin E, vitamin C, vitamin B1, vitamin B2, niacin, niacinamide, pantothenic acid, vitamin B6, vitamin B12, folic acid, biotin, choline, inositol, methionine, calcium, magnesium, potassium, zinc, silicon, manganese, iodine, chromium, and selenium. There are many scientific studies that report positive results in the use of nutrients to eliminate metals and toxins from the body. For more information on nutritional chelation therapies, consult the resources section at the end of this book.

BIOENERGETIC MEDICINE

There are many forms of bioenergetic medicine that are showing promise for brain disorders and for rebalancing the brain's frequencies. The term, "bioenergetic medicine," describes many different forms of natural therapies and techniques, all of which share a common goal of balancing the body's energy systems. While once thought to be esoteric in nature, scientific studies are showing the validity of the energy systems of the body and many of the various forms of healing that help to balance those systems. Some of the therapies include acupuncture and acupressure, quantum biofeedback, energy psychology, and others. First, let me explain some of the primary energy systems in the human body by exploring one of the most ancient forms of bioenergetic medicine: acupuncture.[4]

Acupuncture and Acupressure

Thousands of research studies have proven the healing effects of needling the body in specific locations known as "points" or "acupoints," and millions of people over the last five to ten thousand years, since the advent of acupuncture, have experienced the proof that acupuncture works by witnessing improvements in their symptoms. For those in need of scientific proof, engineers developed instruments called "acupunctuscopes," which prove the existence of the acupuncture points by reading the electrical frequency on the surface of the skin. Changes in electrical frequency occur in the exact location of the acupoints on the body, which are based on ancient texts and drawings.

These points exist in the body in connected lines known as "meridians" or "channels." While many studies had proved the existence of the acupuncture points, until recently scientists still doubted that they were connected.

Over a decade ago, French scientists went to work to prove or disprove the meridian theory. Taking two groups of people, they injected them with radioactive dye. One group was injected with dye in the exact location of the acupuncture points. Participants in the other group were injected in bogus points. The movement of the dye was monitored. Researchers were shocked to discover that where the dye had been injected into real acupuncture points, it flowed in lines in the positions of the meridians recorded by the Chinese millennia ago. Where the dye was injected into bogus points, the dye merely dispersed, without following any lines at all. Numerous other studies have also confirmed the existence of meridians and acupoints in the body.

The World Health Organization endorses acupuncture by publishing a list of dozens of illnesses that acupuncture effectively treats, including headaches and migraines, osteoarthritis, bursitis, tendonitis, sciatica, other musculoskeletal disorders, neurological disorders, and countless others.

The meridians are energy pathways in the body that, when flowing properly, ensure health and vitality. However, when a blockage occurs (which can be caused by any number of things including stress, physical injuries, emotional traumas, allergies, poor nutrition, etc.) the flow of energy is disrupted, and this disruption can cause a multitude of symptoms including pain, inflammation, and virtually any health problem. Energy meridians are similar to a river. If a tree falls in the river, it may disrupt the flow of water through the river and may even affect any tributaries that get their flow of water from the river. A blockage is comparable to the tree, disrupting the proper energy flow throughout the body. The acupressure or acupuncture points are locations along the energy lines where the energy surfaces in the body. These are the locations that the Chinese (and other cultures) documented over five thousand years ago, and whose existence recent research has confirmed. These points have a higher electrical frequency, and respond very well to touch applied in the form of pressure or massage.

In China, acupuncture is practiced widely in hospitals and medical clinics. The West, however, has taken longer to catch on. Perhaps this is due to our experiences with needles, which we associate with large, thick instruments used for drawing blood or delivering vaccinations—the kind that make you jump out of your chair from discomfort or fear. Unlike these needles, acupuncture needles are very fine, much thinner than a pin.

Acupuncture and acupressure have been extensively researched with well over one hundred studies published. Repeatedly, acupuncture and acupressure have been shown to be effective for chronic fatigue syndrome, depression, cognitive impairment, Alzheimer's, and Parkinson's disease. Research shows that acupuncture has improved the clinical symptoms, delayed the progression of the disease, resulted in medication dosage decreases, and reduced drug side effects in Alzheimer's. The use of a form of electro-acupuncture, called transcutaneous electrical nerve stimulation (TENS), has been shown to improve non-verbal, short-term, and long-term memory as well as verbal fluency in patients suffering from early stage Alzheimer's disease.[5] Numerous other studies show the effectiveness of acupuncture on dementia, in studies of both humans and animals.[6]

The many proven beneficial effects of acupuncture warrant its use in most brain disorders. If you just can't stand the thought of needles, give acupressure a try. Most people report that both acupuncture and acupressure are incredibly relaxing and result in more energy as an added bonus to all the other therapeutic effects.

Quantum Biofeedback

Imagine that the latest technology could read stress patterns in your organ systems, structure (bones and cartilage), muscles, hormones, emotional states, blood, energy meridians, and countless other aspects of you that could be underlying factors for disease. What if it also told you about foods that you're eating that are stressing your body as well as those that could improve it? What if it could even inform you about the best possible natural remedies to help you overcome your health concerns? Imagine still that it emitted healing frequencies to your body to help restore health and wellness. Does it all sound too good to be true? Think again. The future of healing has arrived. It's called quantum biofeedback.

Based on the combined principles of acupuncture, homeopathy, quantum physics, and electronics, quantum biofeedback blends the best of ancient eastern thought with modern western technology. According to *Health & Longevity Journal*, "The basis of (quantum biofeedback) technology is the transmission of sixty-five million tiny electromagnetic signals into the body, many times per second. These pulses map the body and its organs and reveal anomalies within the body. The signals feed back to the quantum biofeedback machine and without the patient even being aware of any effect or sensations, the machine calculates a mathematical model based on the voltage, amperage and resistance of the body."

Sometimes our bodies share symptoms to get our attention while the causative factors in disease or illness elude us. That can leave us confused as to which type of natural remedies or therapies would be most beneficial. Quantum biofeedback therapy can provide detailed insight into the myriad factors that affect health.

Quantum biofeedback determines levels of "reactivity" to possible allergens, nutritional deficiencies and excesses and pathogens (viruses, bacteria, fungi, etc.), examines brainwaves, dental concerns, spinal subluxations and other related problems, hormone levels, energy levels, emotions that may be affecting a person's well-being (or lack thereof), organ stress, energy meridian balance, and much more.

Because everyone is unique, understanding what is going on in a person's body is critical to healing. Even the nutritional requirements of people vary as much as seven hundred percent according to Roger Williams, PhD at University of Texas. Most blood tests simply cannot find many nutritional deficiencies, especially those that are subclinical. Yet, even seemingly minor nutritional deficiencies can cause serious damage to a person's health. By having a tool that can find potential problem areas, a person's therapy can be tailored to suit his or her unique needs.

One of the more than one hundred therapies that are part of quantum biofeedback is the allergy and sensitivity program. It screens hundreds of substances to find possible allergens or sensitivities, thereby saving a person from the massive task of weeding them out one by one and potentially sparing him or her years of suffering.

Knowing how emotions are affecting the body is also essential to health. We know that treating someone as merely a physical presence is limiting to his or her possibilities for well-being. By recognizing the person as a mental, emotional, physical, and spiritual person, and then treating them accordingly, the results can be astounding. Quantum biofeedback therapy incorporates all the different facets of healing.

In addition to finding weak areas of a person's health, a quantum biofeedback therapist can also search for harmonious substances that have healing potential for someone. These substances can range from homeopathic remedies, herbs, Bach flower essences, nutritional supplements, and others.

Traditionally, biofeedback systems could only read the results of electro-conductivity tests on the body. In addition to reading the body's functions and dysfunctions, quantum biofeedback can also send harmonious frequencies back to the body to trigger the body's own healing mechanisms to "kick in."

Quantum biofeedback has been used effectively to help balance the underlying bioenergetic imbalances linked with many brain health concerns ranging from toxic overload, depression, learning disabilities, brain hormone imbalances, and brain diseases.

Straps are fastened to the wrists, ankles, and around the forehead. Electrical readings are taken from the body and fed back to the computer for analysis. Acupuncturists have known for thousands of years that these locations on the body have heightened electrical conductivity. Science has since proven this knowledge to be true. What's more, the whole procedure is a totally painless.

Says Noam Friedlander, journalist for *The Times* (London, England), "Complex or not, the results that spew forth on the computer screen will fascinate even the most cynical of visitors."

He explains his review of quantum biofeedback, "After being strapped in myself, it came up with, along with various vitamin deficiencies, a throat infection and a mouth ulcer—I had neither, or so I thought, and the cynic in me left feeling slightly triumphant. The feeling didn't last. The next morning, sure enough, two mouth ulcers had sprung up and a chronic sore throat was starting to develop, which took time and various homeopathic remedies to cure. The machine, once again, had come up trumps."

According to Annie Friedman, a therapist using the machine in London, England, "One woman who came in to have the scan had ever so slightly bulging eyes and the machine came up with three separate readings for thyroid, and when I tested her it showed radiation fallout. Well, it turned out she'd been driving across Europe when Chernobyl went off."

People who have tried quantum biofeedback are often astounded by the incredible accuracy as well as detailed information they receive about their bodies. I was no different the first time I was hooked up for a reading. The machine found detailed information about my health, some of which I (and I alone) knew to be true, but most of it was a powerful learning and healing experience. What amazed me even more so were the improvements I saw in my health following quantum biofeedback therapy. I was hooked, and decided to incorporate quantum biofeedback therapy into my practice.

I believe that Eastern and Western approaches to medicine have the capacity to combine well to form the ultimate in healing experiences. While not a "cure-all" or even touted as a "cure" for brain disease, quantum biofeedback can help a holistic doctor get to the primary imbalances that may be underlying brain disease to assist the body in rebalancing. Unlike pharmaceutical medicine, which focuses primarily on symptom elimination, in the field of natural medicine balance is the ultimate goal.

When choosing a quantum biofeedback therapist it is important to select someone with a background in biofeedback as well as another legitimate health credential. This type of therapy is not just about running the technology—it's about interpretation of the data that will be presented on the computer, which includes nutritional, herbal, homeopathic, disease-related, and other natural medicine data. Your experience is only as valuable as the person behind the machine. The machine is just a tool. Imagine acupuncture needles without a skilled acupuncturist—they'd be useless. Beware of the weekend workshop practitioners—they're plentiful in this field. While they may be well-meaning, you'll probably not get the results you're hoping for unless you see a health practitioner trained at using the quantum biofeedback machine.

There are many excellent natural therapies that offer assistance in the prevention and healing of brain diseases. Choose the one, or ones, that you feel most drawn toward. But, remember, they can only be effective if given adequate time and dedication. Too often, people claim, "I've tried everything," which is not only an exaggeration but also a reflection of their interest in dabbling in, not sticking to, a particular natural therapy. No pharmaceutical drug is effective after only a dose or two. Natural therapies, which typically work on a deeper healing level than just the Band-Aid approach to symptoms drugs provide, can take time and dedication for maximum results.

Maintaining a Healthy Brain for Life

Regardless whether you choose to incorporate natural therapies into your brain health plan, you now have an immensely powerful toolkit at your disposal in the prevention and healing of brain disease: *The Brain Wash* Plan.

For maximum results, be sure to lessen your exposure to harmful neurotoxins as much as possible, eat the wide variety of foods included in *The Brain Wash* Plan, and incorporate many lifestyle suggestions into your daily habits. Brain disease is not an inevitable part of aging. With care and attention to your lifestyle, you can dramatically influence the course your life can take. Remember, you are the director of your life. You can direct it to maximize your genetic potential and live a long and healthy life. I wish you tremendous brain health.

Resources

HEAVY METAL TESTING

Many holistic health professionals offer urine or hair analysis to help you determine the levels of heavy metals like cadmium, aluminum, lead, mercury, and others in your body. Ask your health professional if he/she offers either or both of these tests.

LEAD TEST KITS

The company Pro-Lab sells home test kits for lead on surfaces and lead in water. Call 1–800–427–0550, or visit www.prolabinc.com.

CELLFOOD®

Cellfood is a unique, cell-oxygenating liquid formula that delivers seventy-eight trace minerals, thirty-four enzymes, seventeen amino acids, and electrolytes, and increases the bioavailability of oxygen to the body using a unique water-splitting technology. It is readily absorbed by the body at the cellular level, making a wealth of nutrients available to your cells for optimum healing. Unlike other oxygen products I've tried, Cellfood delivers the oxygen slowly, thereby preventing free radical damage. Cellfood also helps normalize an acidic pH of the body, which is integral to proper detoxification and healing. It also assists with energy and boosts the immune system. I recommend taking eight drops of Cellfood three times per day in a glass of pure water or juice. In addition to oxygen, it contains the following essential nutrients.

1. Trace Minerals: actinium, antimony, argon, astatine, barium, beryllium, bismuth, boron, bromine, calcium, carbon, cerium, cesium, chromium, cobalt, copper, dysprosium, erbium, europium, fluorine, gadolinium, gallium, germanium, gold, hafnium, helium, holmium, hydrogen, indium, iodine, iridium, iron, krypton, lanthanum, lithium, lutetium, magnesium, manganese, molybdenum, neodymium, neon, nickel, niobium, nitrogen, osmium, oxygen, palladium, phosphorous, platinum, polonium, potassium, praseodymium, promethium, rhenium, rhodium, rubidium, ruthenium, samarium, selenium, silica, silicon, silver, sodium, sulfur, tantalum, technetium, tellurium, terbium, thallium, thorium, tin, titanium, tungsten, vanadium, xenon, ytterbium, zinc, and zirconium (does not contain aluminium, cadmium, chlorine, mercury, lead, or radium).
2. Metabolic Enzymes: hydrolases, carbohydrases (maltase, sucrase); emulsin nucleases (polynucleotidase, nucleotidase); hydrases (fumarase, enolase); peptidases (aminopolypeptidase, dipeptidase, prolinase); copper enzymes (tyrosinase, ascorbic acid oxidase); esterase (lipase, phosphotase, sulphatase); iron enzymes (catalase, cytochrome oxidase, peroxidase); enzymes containing coenzymes 1 and/or 2 (lactic dehydrogenase, robison ester dehydrogenase); yellow enzymes (Warburg's yellow enzymes, diaphorase, Haas enzyme, cytochrome C reductase); enzymes which reduce cytochrome (succinic dehydrogenase); aidase (urease); mutases (aldehyde mutase, glyoxalase); desmolases (zymohexase, carboxylase); and other enzymes (phosphorylase, phosphohexisomerase, hexokinase, phosphoglumutase).
3. Amino Acids: alanine, arginine, aspartic acid, cystine, glutamic acid, glycine, histidine, isoleucine, lysine, methionine, phenylalanine, proline, serine, threonine, tryptophan, tyrosine, and valine.

Cellfood is available from most health food stores and health-care practitioners. For more information contact Lumina Health Products at www.luminahealth.com or 1–800–749–9196 or e-mail info@luminahealth.com.

Organic and Natural Mattresses and Bedding

Sleeptek is a manufacturer/retailer of a range of organic and natural bedding options, including organic cotton mattresses, natural rubber mattresses and pillows, organic buckwheat pillows, organic cotton mattress toppers, and organic comforters. They do not use any toxic materials during the manufacturing of their bedding products, and they are completely free of toxic flame retardants. The company routinely ships throughout North America, but shipping to other countries is also possible. Their main organic bedding line is called Obasan. Visit www.sleeptek.ca or www.obasan.ca

Sleeptek
50 Colonnade Road,
Ottawa, ON K2E 7J6
1-866-603-5556
613–727–5537

More Brain Information

Additional information on the brain, the natural treatment of brain disease, and the blood-brain barrier can be found in two excellent books:

The BrainGate: The Little-Known Doorway That Lets Nutrients In and Keeps Toxic Agents Out
By J. Robert Hatherill, PhD

ISBN: 0-898526-141-3
LifeLine Press
One Massachusetts Avenue, NW
Washington, DC 20001
www.lifelinepress.com
202–216–0600

BrainRecovery.com: Powerful Therapy for Challenging Brain Disorders
By David Perlmutter, MD

ISBN: 0-9635874-1-2
The Perlmutter Health Center
800 Goodlett Road North, Suite 270
Naples, FL 34102
www.perlhealth.com
239–649–7400

BrainRecovery.com is also an excellent resource for information on Hyperbaric Oxygen Therapy (HBOT).

WATER FILTRATION

There are many excellent manufacturers of water filtration products. One of the easiest to access is through Nikken at www.nikken.com.

Alternatively, visit www.5pillars.com to learn more about water filtration options. To help you select the right system for you, contact: Murray Smith and Rita Maccagno-Smith at bushmom@telusplanet. net. Mention ID #791562500 when purchasing.

MEDITATION AND STRESS MANAGEMENT

My favourite book to help you learn how to meditate:

Meditation for Wimps: Finding Your Balance in an Imperfect World
By Miriam Austin

ISBN: 0-806969-17-2
Sterling Publishing, Inc.
387 Park Avenue South
New York, NY 10016
www.sterlingpublishing.com
212–532–7160

BIOENERGETIC MEDICINE

For more information about Bioenergetic Medicine, consult these
excellent books:

*The Promise of Energy Psychology: Revolutionary Tools for Dramatic
Personal Change*
By David Feinstein, Donna Eden and Gary Craig

ISBN: 1-58542-442-0
375 Hudson Street
New York, NY 10014
www.penguingroup.com
212–366–2636

This book includes some excellent information, including photographs
of some brain scans before and after treatment using the energy psychology methods outlined in the book.

Energy Medicine
By Donna Eden and David Feinstein

ISBN: 1-585420-21-2
375 Hudson Street
New York, NY 10014
www.penguingroup.com
212–366–2636

Both books and additional information are also available through www.innersource.net.

QUANTUM BIOFEEDBACK

For more information on quantum biofeedback, visit www.EnergyEffect.com, click on "Articles," and select "A Quantum Leap in Healing."

DETOXIFICATION THERAPY

For more information about detoxifying your whole body, and a unique systematic approach to improving the functioning of all your detox organs, including intestines, urinary tract, liver, gallbladder, lymphatic system, skin, respiratory system, and blood, check out:

The 4-Week Ultimate Body Detox Plan: A Program for Greater Energy, Health and Vitality
By Michelle Schoffro Cook, DNM, DAc, CNC

    ISBN: 0-471-79213-6
    John Wiley & Sons, Canada, Ltd.
    22 Worcester Road
    Etobicoke, ON M9W 1L1
    www.wiley.com
    416–236–4433

NUTRITIONAL CHELATION

Creative Nutrition Canada Corporation sells a nutritional chelation formula called Vitamost RTRE. For more information or to purchase this product, contact:

    Creative Nutrition Canada Corporation
    PO Box 99
    Parry Sound, ON P2A 2X2

1–800–841–2288
www.cncvitamost.com

Mention referral ID#11512 to set up a Preferred Customer account. There is a small fee that allows you to purchase product and obtain a discount on them.

ORAGACYN P-73

To purchase this product or obtain more information about it, visit www.p-73.com.

VACCINES AND IMMUNIZATION

For a comprehensive review of the many issues related to immunization, read this excellent book:

Immunization: History, Ethics, Law and Health
By Catherine J. M. Diodati

ISBN: 0-968508-00-6
Integral Aspects Inc.
5060 Tecumseh Road East, Suite 439
Windsor, ON N8T 1C1
519–972–9567

HOLISTIC DENTISTRY

For more information about mercury amalgam dental fillings and the correct removal of them, check out the following book or the Holistic Dental Association's website, www.holisticdental.org.

Uninformed Consent: The Hidden Dangers in Dental Care
By Hal A. Huggins and Thomas E. Levy

ISBN: 1-57174-11-78
Hampton Roads Publishing Company
1125 Stoney Ridge Road
Charlottesville, VA 22902
www.hamptonroadspub.com
1–800–660–2662

Fish Oil Supplements and Lead-free Calcium Supplements

Metagenics manufactures fish oil supplements that are free from toxic ingredients like mercury and PCBs. The company also conducts third-party laboratory testing of its calcium supplements, which consistently are devoid of measurable amounts of lead. The supplements are only sold to holistic health practitioners and some natural pharmacies, so you may need to visit your local health practitioner to purchase these products. Unfortunately, I am not familiar with other supplement manufacturers that offer fish oil and calcium supplements, verified by third-party testing to be non-contaminated. For more information about their products, visit www.metagenics.com. The company also offers information on their website for people trying to find health care practitioners who sell Metagenics products (under the "Contact" link).

Far-Infrafred Sauna

There is a vast range of saunas on the market, ranging from ineffective and poorly constructed, to high quality, therapeutic ones. For more information visit www.infraredsauna.net to learn about infrared saunas for detoxification, healing and pain relief.

Endnotes

INTRODUCTION

1. "Live Well, Resist Alzheimer's." Medical News Today http://www.medicalnewstoday.com/medicalnews.php?newsid=11003.
2. Alan C. Logan, ND, FRSH, *The Brain Diet* (Nashville, TN: Cumberland House, 2006), 1.
3. Rachael Moeller Gorman, "Food for Thought: Can healthy eating help your brain stay sharp?" *Eating Well*, April/May 2006.

CHAPTER 1

1. Ronald Kotulak, *Inside the Brain: Revolutionary Discoveries of How the Mind Works* (Kansas City, MO: Andrews McMeel Publishing, 1997), 17.
2. Ibid., xi.
3. Ibid., 5.
4. Ibid., 133.
5. J. Robert Hatherhill, PhD, *The BrainGate: the Little-Known Doorway that Lets Nutrients In and Keeps Toxic Agents Out* (Washington, DC: Lifeline Press, 2003), 9.
6. Ibid., 12.

CHAPTER 2

1. Richard H. Casdorph and Morton Walker, *Toxic Metal Syndrome: How Metal Poisonings Can Affect Your Brain* (Garden City Park, NY: Avery Publishing Group, 1995),185.

2. Ibid.,187.
3. William H. Philpott, MD and Dwight K. Kalita, PhD, *Brain Allergies: The Psychonutrient and Magnetic Connections* (Los Angeles, CA: Keats Publishing, 2000), 68–69.
   Hatherhill, 147.
   Kylie Taggart, "Calcium supplements may have lead risk," *The Medical Post*, October 24, 2000, Volume 36, Issue 36.
   Nutritional Tests (Innisfail, AB: Professional Health Products),14–15.
   David W. Rowland, PhD, RNC, *Advanced Nutri-Body® Analysis* (Parry Sound, ON: Creative Nutrition Canada, 1999).
4. Hatherhill, 35.
5. Casdorph and Walker, 187.
6. Ibid., 188–189.
7. Ibid., 188.
8. Rachael Moeller Gorman, "Food for Thought: Can healthy eating help your brain stay sharp?" *Eating Well*, April/May 2006.
9. David Perlmutter, MD, FANC and Carol Colman, *The Better Brain Book* (New York, NY: Riverhead Books, 2004), 28.
10. Hatherhill, 133.
11. Ibid.,19.
12. Perlmutter and Colman, 56.
13. Ibid., 150.
14. Hatherhill, 149.
15. Ibid.,129.
16. Philpott and Kalita, 68–69.
    Hatherhill, 147.
    Taggart.
    Nutritional Tests, 14–15.
    Rowland.
17. Ibid., 68–69.
18. Perlmutter and Colman, 150.
19. Hatherhill, 36.
20. Ibid., 32.
21. Ibid., 32.

22. Philpott and Kalita, 68–69.
   Hatherhill, 32, 35–36, 147.
   Taggart.
   Nutritional Tests, 14–15.
   Rowland.
23. Ibid., 68–69.
24. Hatherhill, 33.
24. Pro-Lab Inc., "Lead in Water." Pro-Lab http://www.prolabinc.com/products.asp?kit=leadinwater.
26. Taggart.
27. Mercola, MD and Klinghardt, MD, "Mercury Toxicity and Systemic Elimination Agents," *Journal of Nutritional and Environmental Medicine*, March 2001.
28. Perlmutter and Colman, 146.
29. Hatherhill, 133.
30. Ibid, 34.
31. Ibid., 34.
32. Perlmutter and Colman146.
33. Gary Null, PhD, *The Complete Encyclopedia of Natural Healing* (New York, NY: Kensington Publishing Corp., 2005), 81.
34. Mercola and Klinghardt.
35. Ibid.
36. Philpott and Kalita, 68–69.
   Hatherhill, 32, 35–36, 147.
   Taggart.
   Nutritional Tests, 14–15.
   Rowland.
37. Philpott and Kalita, 68–69.
38. Perlmutter and Colman, 148.
39. Ibid., 147.
40. Mercola and Klinghardt.
41. Ibid.
42. Perlmutter and Colman, 148.
43. Mercola and Klinghardt.
44. Ibid.

45. "Dental Amalgam Controversy." Wikipedia http://en.wikipedia. org/wiki/Dental_amalgam_controversy.

46. Ibid.

47. Ibid.

48. Mercola and Klinghardt.

49. Perlmutter and Colman, 147.

50. Mercola, MD. "Calculate Your Child's Risk of Mercury Poisoning from Vaccines." Mercola http://www.mercola.com/2005/apr/23/ mercury_poison.htm.

51. Mercola and Klinghardt.

52. Ibid.

CHAPTER 3

1. Juliette Jowit, "Pollutants Cause Huge Rise in Brain Diseases," *The Observer*, UK News, August 15, 2004.

2. Ibid.

3. Ibid.

4. Ibid.

5. Francesca Lymn, "Our bodies, Our Landfills?" *MSNBC*, November 4, 2003.

6. "Do You Have the Right Tools to Address Your Patients' Detoxification Needs?" *MetaNews*, May 1, 2006.

7. Lymn.

8. Jacqueline Krohn and Frances Taylor, *Natural Detoxification: A Practical Encyclopedia* (Port Roberts, WA: Hartley & Marks Publishers, Inc., 2000).

9. "Detoxification." Informational Brochure. (Advanced Nutrition Publications, Inc., 1994).

10. David E. Root and Joan Anderson, "Reducing Toxic Body Burdens Advancing in Innovative Technique," *Occupational Health and Safety News Digest 2*, April 1986.

11. Hatherhill, 30.

12. *MetaNews*.

13. Richard Mesquita. "Pesticide and Herbicide Contamination." Mercola http://www.mercola.com.

14. "Pesticides." Pro-Lab http://www.prolabinc.com/products. asp?kit=pesticides
15. Mesquita.
16. Ibid.
17. Doris J. Rapp, MD, *Our Toxic World: A Wake Up Call: Chemicals Damage Your Body, Brain, Behaviour and Sex* (Buffalo, NY: Environmental Medical Research Foundation, 2004).
18. Ibid., 319.
19. Mesquita.
20. Daniella Brower. "Children Face Danger in the Schoolyard Grass from Pesticides." CNN.com http://www.cnn.com. March 2, 2000.
21. Ibid.
22. Ibid.
23 Environmental News Network staff. "We're Poisoning Our Kids, toxins report says." CNN.com http://www.cnn.com September 11, 2000.
24. Organic Consumers Association, "Pesticides causing brain damage," *Organic Bytes*, April 14, 2003.
25. Michelle Schoffro Cook, DNM, DAc, CNC, *The 4-Week Ultimate Body Detox Plan* (Toronto, ON: John Wiley & Sons Canada, Ltd., 2004).
26. "Health Impacts: Pesticides." Clean Air http://www.cseindia. org/html/lab/health_pest.htm.
27. "British Scientists Study Link Between Pesticides and Parkinson's." Reuters Health. http://www.reutershealth.com May 17, 2002.
28. "Home and Garden Pesticides Increase Parkinson's Risk," *American Academy of Neurology's 52nd Annual Meeting*, May 2000.
29. "Pesticide Combination Linked to Parkinson's," *Journal of Neuroscience 2000*, (Volume 20, 2000), 9207–9214.
30. "Yet more pesticides linked to Parkinson's." Reuters Health. http://www.reutershealth.com. November 13, 2003.
31. The Associated Press. "Traces of Fire Retardant Found in Salmon: Traces of Industrial-Strength Fire Retardant Found in Salmon

Around the World, Study Says." ABC News http://www.abc-NEWS.com. August 10, 2004.

32. Martin Mittelstaedt, "Ottawa Plans to Snuff Out Flame Retardants," *The Globe and Mail*, May 30, 2006.

33. Ibid.

34. "Flame Retardants Found on Supermarket Shelves," *American Chemical Society*, September 8, 2004.

35. Ibid.

36. Ibid.

37. "PBDEs—The New Global Toxins," Labour Environmental Alliance Society.

38. Pravin Char, "Ritalin 'May Cause Damage to bBrains,'" *ThisisLondon*, December 17, 2003.

39. Dan Olmsted, "The Age of Autism: A pretty big secret," *UPI*, December 7, 2005.

40. Jonathan D. Rockoff, "New life seen for vaccine industry," *Baltimore Sun*, June 6, 2006.

41. Ibid.

42. Rose Marie Williams. "Fragrance Alters Mood and Brain Chemistry - Health Risks and Environmental Issues." The Townsend Letter for Doctors and Patients http://www.findarticles.com/p/articles/mi_m0ISW/is_249/ai_114820660/print. 2004.

43. Ibid.

CHAPTER 4

1. Carol Simontacci, *The Crazy Makers: How the Food Industry Is Destroying Our Brains and Harming Our Children* (New York, NY: Tarcher Penguin, 2000).

2. Ibid.

3. "Epilepsy drug helps fight Parkinson's," *Neurology*, April 24, 2000.

4. Fitzgerald, 73.

5. Schoffro Cook.

6. Ibid.
7. Ibid.
8. Schoffro Cook.
9. Nancy Appleton, *Lick the Sugar Habit* (New York, NY: Avery Publishing Group, 1996).
   Lynne Melcombe, *Health Hazards of White Sugar* (Vancouver, BC: Alive Books, 2001).
10. Ibid.
11. Hatherhill, 81.
12. Ibid., 81.
13. Ibid., 82.
14. "The Importance of Detoxification," Informational Brochure. (Advanced Nutrition Publications, Inc., 2002).
15. Fitzgerald, 70.
   Jacqueline Krohn, MD and Frances Taylor, MA, *Natural Detoxification: A Practical Encyclopedia* (Port Roberts, WA: Hartley & Marks Publishers, Inc. 2000), 115.
16. Schoffro Cook.

CHAPTER 5

1. Schoffro Cook.
2. Ibid.
3. "Getting to the Root of the Problem: Part 3—Dysbiosis." Food-allergy.org http://www.food-allergy.org/root3.html.
4. Xandria Williams, *The Herbal Detox Plan* (Carlsbad, CA: Hay House, 2004), 82.
5. Logan.
6. Ibid., 116.
7. Ibid., 118.
8. Schoffro Cook.

CHAPTER 6

1. Julia Tolliver Maranan, "The Right Nutrients to Age-Proof Your Brain," *Natural Health*, April 2003.

2. Joseph Mercola, MD. "Keep Alzheimer's Away with Fish Oil's Secret Weapon." Mercola http://www.mercola.com. April 6, 2005.
3. James Balch, MD, and Mark Stengler, ND, *Prescription for Natural Cures* (Hoboken, NJ: John Wiley & Sons, Inc., 2004.) 36.
4. Tolliver Maranan.
5. Ibid.
6. Ibid.
7. George Mateljan. "'Olives' The World's Healthiest Foods." The World's Healthiest Foods http://www.whfoods.com
8. "Tryptophan, Niacin Protect Against Alzheimer's." Reuters Health http://www.reutershealth.com.
9. Tolliver Maranan.
10. Ibid.
11. Genevieve Des Jarlais. "Alternatives to Prozac." Alternative Medicine http://www.AlternativeMedicine.com.
12. Tolliver Maranan.
13. Ibid.
14. "Autism." Alive http://www.alive.com.
15. Rachael Moeller Gorman, "Food for Thought: Can healthy eating help your brain stay sharp?" *Eating Well*, April/May 2006.
16. Tolliver Maranan.
17. Ibid.
18. Ibid.
19. Jill Hillhouse, RNCP, "Zinc and Selenium," *alive*, June 2006,. 60–61.
20. Hatherhill, 150.
21. Ibid., 88–89.
22. Ibid., 89.
23. Ibid., 89.
24. "Red wine molecule may protect brain from Alzheimer's." Reuters Health http://www.reutershealth.com, December 31, 2003.
25. Kathleen Barnes, "Preserve Memory," *alive*, June 2006, 89.
26. "Cigarettes, Tea, and Cola Linked to Lower Risk of Parkinson's,"

American Journal of Epidemiology, 2002 (Volume 155), 732–738.

27. "Coffee Lowers Risk of Parkinson's," *Journal of the American Medical Association,* May 24/31, 2000.

28. Moeller Gorman.

29. Hatherhill, 88.

30. Barbara Hustedt Crook, "Guilt-free Indulgence," *Woman's World,* Feb 15, 2005.

31. "Anti-inflammatory Drugs Dramatically Reduce Parkinson's Risk," *Archive of Neurology,* 2003 (Volume 60),1059–1064.

32. Michelle Schoffro Cook, DNM, DAc, CNC, *Healing Injuries the Natural Way* (Toronto, ON: Your Health Press, Inc., 2004), 29.

33. Ibid.

34. George Mateljan. "The World's Healthiest Foods: Onions." The World's Healthiest Foods http://www.whfoods.com/genpage.php?tname=foodspice&dbid=45.

35. George Mateljan. "The World's Healthiest Foods: Kidney Beans." The World's Healthiest Foods hhttp://www.whfoods.com/genpage.php?tname=foodspice&dbid=87.

36. David Perlmutter, MD, *BrainRecovery.com: Powerful Therapy for Challenging Brain Disorders*, (Naples, FL: The Perlmutter Health Center, 2000), 6.

37. Ibid., 6.

38. "Coenzyme Q10 Slows Progression of Parkinson's," *Archives of Neurology*, 2002 (Volume 59),1541–1550.

39. Ibid.

40. "Alzheimer's Linked to Mitochondrial Mutations." Wired News www.wired.com/news/medtech/0,1286,64107,00.html?tw=wn_tophead_9.

41. Dr. Mercola. "Chlorella – A Natural Wonder Food." Mercola http://www.mercola.com.

42. Perlmutter, *BrainRecovery.com*, 7.

43. Balch and Stengler, 562.

44. Meg Lundstrom, "7 Easy Ways to Feel Happier Now!" *Woman's*

World, September 19, 2006, 12.

45. Kathleen Barnes, "The Little Fiber Pill that Can Detox Your Whole Body," *Woman's World,* April 27, 2004. 24.

46. Ann Louise Gittleman, MS, CNS, *The Fat Flush Plan* (New York, NY: McGraw-Hill, 2002), 35.

47. Ibid. 19.

48. Ibid, 35.

49. Ibid. 42.

50. Carol Simontacci, *The Crazy Makers: How the Food Industry Is Destroying Our Brains and Harming Our Children* (New York, NY: Tarcher Penguin, 2000).

51. Ibid.

52. Ibid.

53. Ibid.

54. Ibid.

CHAPTER 7

1. "Sage May Help Alzheimers Sufferers." Independent http://www. independent.co.uk. August 29, 2003.

2. Peter J. Houghton, B. Pharm, PhD, "Activity and Constituents of Sage Relevant to the Potential Treatment of Symptoms of Alzheimer's Disease," *Herbalgram: The Journal of the American Botanical Council,* Number 61, 2004.

3. "Sage May Help Alzheimers Sufferers." The Independent. www. independent.co.uk. August 29, 2003.

4. Houghton.

5. Moeller Gorman.

6. "Curry Ingredient May Stop Alzheimer's." Medical News Today http://www.medicalnewstoday.com/medicalnews. php?newsid=13116.

7. Michael Colgan, PhD. "Save Your Brain." Vista http://www. vistamagonline.com/articles.

8. Schoffro Cook, *Healing.*

9. "The Brain Food Herb." Self Help Daily http://selfhelpdaily. com/herbs-that-boost-brainpower-part-4.

10. Maria Noel Mandile, "Vinpocetine," *Natural Health Magazine*, January/February 2002.
11. Ibid.
12. Ibid.
13. Ibid.
14. Perlmutter, *BrainRecovery.com*.
15. Michael Murray, ND, *Dr. Murray's Total Body Tune-Up* (New York, NY: Bantam Books, 2000).
16. Balch and Stengler, 37.
17. Dr. Cass Ingram. "Amyotrophic Lateral Sclerosis (Lou Gehrig's Disease)." North American Herb & Spice www.p-73.com.
18. George Mateljan. "The World's Healthiest Foods: Rosemary." The World's Healthiest Foods www.whfoods.com/genpage. php?tname=foodspice&dbid=75.
19. Ibid.
20. Ibid.
21. Ibid.
22. Murray, 253.
23. *International Journal of Sport Nutrition and Exercise Metabolism*, June 2006.
24. "Tai Chi and Yohimbine Could Help Parkinsons" www.reuter-shealth.com November 13, 2002.
25. Schoffro Cook, *Ultimate Body*.
26. Ibid.
27. Ibid.
28. Ibid.
29. Frances Albrecht, MS, CN, "The Basics of Detoxing Your Liver," *Healthwell*, April 1997.
30. Sandra Cabot, MD, *The Liver Cleansing Diet* (SCB International, Inc., 2000), 69.
31. "Are You Taking the Life Out of Your Liver?" Great American Products http://www.greatamericanproducts.com.
32. Williams, 129.
33. Cabot, 68.
34. Gittleman, 19–20.
35. Albrecht.

36. Schoffro Cook, *Ultimate Body.*

CHAPTER 8

1. Kevin Eikenberry. "Re-Energize Your Brain." The Mental Fitness Center http://thementalfitnesscenter.com/reenergizeyourbrain.html.

2. Barbara Hustedt Crook, "Guilt-free Indulgence," *Woman's World,* Feb 15, 2005.

3. Ibid.

4. "Massage benefits Parkinsons Sufferers." Ivanhoe's Medical Breakthroughs http://www.ivanhoe.com. October 19, 2001.

5. "Tai Chi and Yohimbine Could Help Parkinson's." Reuters Health http://www.reutershealth.com. November 13, 2002.

6. "Study sheds light on how education may prevent Alzheimer's." Reuters Health http://www.reutershealth.com. August 7, 2003.

7. Ibid.

8. "5 Ways to keep your brain in shape!" *Woman's World,* March 7, 2006, 39.

9. "Sun Exposure Decreases Risk of MS." Mercola http://www.mercola.com. August 27, 2003.

10. Ibid.

11. Ibid.

12. Hustedt Crook.

13. "Depression Triples Risk of Parkinson's" *Neurology 2002* (Volume 58),1501–1504.

14. Ibid.

15. "Brain Scans, Blood Tests Show Positive Effects of Meditation," *Health Behavior News Service,* August 16, 2003.

16. Tim Htut. "The Effects of Meditation on the Body." Nibbana http://www.*Triplegem.plus.com.* September 18, 1999

17. Schoffro Cook, *Ultimate Body.*

18. "Love is a Drug." Mercola http://www.mercola.com. February 14, 2006.

CHAPTER 9

1. Brain Research Centre at the University of British Columbia. "Neurodegneration." Brain Research Centre http://www.brain. ubc.ca/neurodegeneration.htm. 2003.
2. Perlmutter, *BrainRecovery.com.*
3. Ibid., 73.
4. Brain Research Centre.
5. Perlmutter, *BrainRecovery.com*, 70.
6. Ibid., 71.
7. Ibid., 72.
8. Ibid., 74.
9. Ibid., 74.
10. Balch and Stengler, 35.
11. Ibid. 38.
12. Ibid. 38.
13. Ibid., 68.
14. Ibid., 71.
15. "Brain Inflammation Link to Autism." BBC News http://news. bbc.co.uk/2/hi/health/4004075.stm. November 15, 2004.
16. Ibid., 81.
17. Ibid., 81.
18. BBC News.
19. Ibid.
20. "Autism." Alive.com http://www.alive.com
21. Ibid.
22. Ibid.
23. Ibid.
24. Logan, 22.
25. Balch and Stengler, 182.
26. Karin Evans. "Brain Food: The Natural Cure for Depression." Alternative Medicine.com http://www.AlternativeMedicine. com.
27. Patrick Casanova. "Multiple Chemical Sensitivity: A Literary Critique." Environmental Illness Resource http://www.ei-resource.org/Articles/mcs-art04.asp.

28. Andrew Weil, MD. "The Mystery of Multiple Chemical Sensitivity." Dr. Andrew Weil's Self-Healing http://www.drweilselfhealing.com. April 2004.
29. Casanova.
30. Ibid.
31. Murray.
32. Balch and Stengler,. 409.
33. Perlmutter, *BrainRecovery.com*, 13.
34. Ibid., 14.
35. Ibid., 14.
36. Murray.
37. Balch and Stengler, 486.
38. Ibid., 488.
39. Perlmutter, *BrainRecovery.com*, 145.
40. Kathleen Barnes, "The Little Fiber Pill That Can Detox Your Whole Body," *Woman's World*, April 27, 2004, 24.
41. Schoffro Cook, *Ultimate Body*.
42. Tutti Gould DC, ND and Michelle Decary, "Homeopathic Detox" *HNV: Health 'N Vitality*, May 2006.

CHAPTER 10

1. Schoffro Cook, *Ultimate Body*.
2. Perlmutter, *BrainRecovery.com*.
3. Rose Marie Williams, "Fragrance alters mood and brain chemistry – Health Risks and Environmental Issues," *Townsend Letter for Doctors and Patients*, 2004.
4. Michelle Schoffro Cook, *Healing Injuries*.
5. Y. Guo, X. Shi, H. Uchiyama, A. Hasegawa, Y. Nakagawa, M. Tanaka, and I. Fukumoto, "A study on the rehabilitation of cognitive function and short-term memory in patients with Alzheimer's disease using transcutaneous electrical nerve stimulation," *Frontiers of Medical and Biological Engineering*, Volume 11, Issue 4 (Nagaoka, Japan: Institute of Biomedical Engineering, Nagaoka University of Technology, 2002), 237–247.

6. J. Yu, C. Liu, X. Zhang, and J. Han, "Acupuncture improved cognitive impairment caused by multi-infact dementia in rats," *Physiology and Behaviour*, November 15, 2005.

Index

ABOUT *the* Author

Michelle Schoffro Cook, DNM, DAc, CNC, CITP, is the bestselling author of *The 4-Week Ultimate Body Detox Plan*, a doctor of natural medicine, doctor of acupuncture, holistic life coach®, biofeedback therapist, holistic nutritionist, energy medicine practitioner, Reconnective™ healing practitioner, and Reiki Master. Dr. Michelle Schoffro Cook's regular columns and contributions appear in the popular health magazines, *Health 'N Vitality, SpaLife, Wellbeing Journal,* and *Herbs for Health.* She has contributed over three hundred articles to more than sixty magazines, journals, and newspapers worldwide and is a popular biweekly guest on CBC Radio's *Wildrose Country.*

Your Health Press released Dr. Schoffro Cook's second book, *Healing Injuries the Natural Way*, in early 2004 (www.healinginjuries.com). She is the recipient of numerous awards, including the prestigious *Forty Under 40 Award* as one of the top business people and leaders in Canada's Capital Region under the age of forty, and a *World Leading Intellectual Award* for her contribution to the advancement of natural medicine. Dr. Schoffro Cook has also received four communications and writing awards for her work. She works and lives with her husband in beautiful British Columbia, Canada. For more information on her work visit www.EnergyEffect.com or www.DrMichelleCook.com.